MW01528279

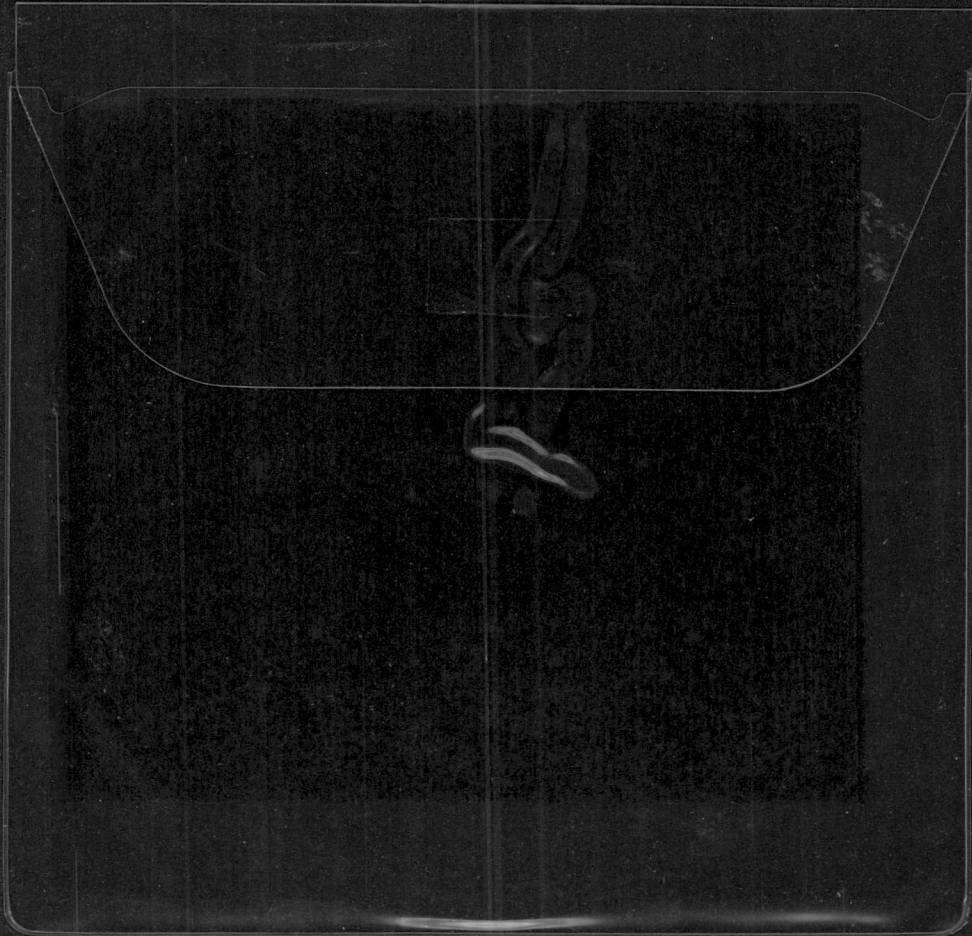

Atlas of
Cataract Surgery

System requirement:
- **Windows XP or above**
- **Power DVD player (Software)**
- **Windows media player 10.0 version or above**
- **Quick time player version 6.5 or above**

Accompanying DVD ROM is playable only in Computer and not in DVD player.

Kindly wait for few seconds for DVD to autorun. If it does not autorun then please do the following:
- Click on my computer
- Click the **drive labelled JAYPEE** and after opening the drive, kindly double click the file **Jaypee**

DVD Contents

Atlas of
Cataract Surgery

K Ravi Kumar Reddy MS DO
Professor and Head of the Department
Department of Ophthalmology
Osmania Medical College
Sarojini Devi Eye Hospital
Hyderabad (India)

P Satyavani MS DO
Assistant Professor
Department of Ophthalmology
Osmania Medical College
Sarojini Devi Eye Hospital
Hyderabad (India)

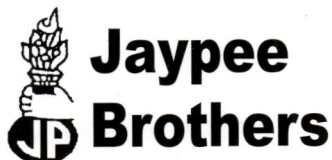

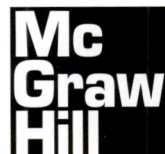

Jaypee
Brothers

Mc Graw Hill Medical

© 2009, Jaypee Brothers Medical Publishers
First published in India in 2009 by
Jaypee Brothers Medical Publishers (P) Ltd.

Corporate Office
4838/24 Ansari Road, Daryaganj, **New Delhi** - 110002, India, +91-11-43574357

Registered Office
B-3 EMCA House, 23/23B Ansari Road, Daryaganj, **New Delhi** 110 002, India
Phones: +91-11-23272143, +91-11-23272703, +91-11-23282021,
+91-11-23245672, Rel: +91-11-32558559 Fax: +91-11-23276490, +91-11-23245683
e-mail: jaypee@jaypeebrothers.com, Website: www.jaypeebrothers.com

First published in USA by The McGraw-Hill Companies, 2 Penn Plaza, New York, NY 10121.
Exclusively worldwide distributor except South Asia (India, Nepal, Sri Lanka, Bhutan, Pakistan, Bangladesh, Malaysia).

ISBN-13: 978-0-07-163445-8
ISBN-10: 0-07-163445-2

To

My Parents and Family Members

Foreword

Ophthalmology entered its golden period and continues to be in it ever since Prof. Harold Ridley invented IOL implantation. All of us have seen a sea of changes taking place in the art of cataract surgery in last 2 decades.

Indian surgeons have earned a great respect internationally for their surgical skills and innovations. The backlog of cataract blindness in our country has been so successfully tackled by our surgeons and NGOs that our volume practice is appreciated by all. We are the world leaders in this aspect and many countries look up to us to guide them and train them in this regard.

Most of us in our country have to play a dual role of running a private clinic and do some community outreach programme. Hence naturally it is necessary to keep a perfect blend of SICS and Phaco in our practice.

It is indeed a task keeping track of all the new innovations happening in the technology of the machine and procedures. Very often when you have learnt and mastered one step or procedure its time for learning a new one. Taking all these things into consideration Dr. Ravi Kumar Reddy for whom I have greatest respect as a good clinician, administrator and a fine human being, has come out with an excellent Atlas on Cataract Surgery which is specially aimed at helping upcoming ophthalmologist and ophthalmology in transition.

There are books of such types written by foreign authors, but what is important is that this book is written by one of us and it is easy for us to relate to his way of thinking.

He is fully aware of ground realities and the type of difficulties doctor faces in his/her stressful transition.

Dr. Reddy has taken pains to look at this subject from all the angles so as to make it useful and practical. I congratulate him on taking up this important task in spite of his tight schedule to help postgraduates and ophthalmologists in transition.

Finally I strongly recommend this book to anybody who wants to improve his cataract surgery.

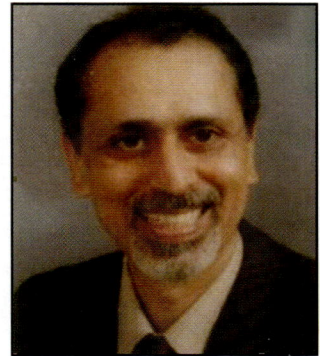

Suhas Haldipurkar

Preface

This book is a guide to budding cataract surgeons particularly the postgraduate students and upcoming ophthalmic surgeons, as this book mainly deals with the practical aspects of present day cataract surgery with photographic and diagrammatic illustrations. We also tried to include some of the special situations in which cataract surgery would be a challenge to the upcoming surgeons. The recent advances in cataract surgery were also described in brief at the end.

In this atlas of cataract surgery we have dealt with the various aspects of SICS and phacoemulsification. In section-1 we have discussed briefly about preoperative evaluation, operating room setup, some of the aspects in cataract surgery in common for SICS and phacoemulsification.

In section-2 different methods of SICS have been described with the necessary photographs and diagrams

In section-3 some of the practical tips have been mentioned for surgeons beginning phacoemulsification after they are well versed with SICS. The phacoemulsifier and the various techniques of nucleus management in phacoemulsification have been described.

In section-4 cataract surgery in special situations , the important complications of cataract surgery and their management are dealt with. A brief mention of the recent advances in cataract surgery has been made in this section.

We would like to update this atlas as and when required in the future editions. We would like to sincerely advice the readers to follow this book as a practical guide and go through the other available books for more detailed information about the topics of their interest .

We are giving a DVD of the necessary surgical videos along with the book.

K Ravi Kumar Reddy
P Satyavani

Acknowledgements

We would like to sincerely thank all our colleagues and our postgraduate students of Sarojini Devi eye hospital, for extending their support in writing this book. We thank our postgraduate students Dr. Thandava Krishna, Dr. Venugopal Reddy and Dr. Jayavani for their help in bringing out this book. Our thanks to Dr. Rupak Kumar Reddy who helped us taking the videos and photographs necessary for the book.

We thank the staff of Medivision eye care center for extending their support.

Finally we are grateful to our beloved family members for extending their valuable support in completing this book.

Contents

SECTION - 5 Complications

Introduction

Cataract surgery is one of the most commonest surgeries performed on the human body. Modern methods of surgery give early rehabilitation, stable refraction and well centered intraocular lens.

The idea of presenting this color atlas is, to provide a practical approach to sutureless cataract surgery and to deal with special situations and complications of cataract surgery. Sutureless cataract surgery can be done by manual technique (SICS) or by use of a phacoemulsifier. Phacoemulsification is definitely advantageous, but in view of a long learning curve, the more prohibitive cost factor and the backlog of cataract cases, even the manual SICS is needed in the present scenario.

In this atlas we have illustrated the initial approach for both procedures in a combined fashion. The nucleus management is illustrated separately according to the procedure. We have also touched upon frequently encountered complications and special situations and suggested corrective practical measures with illustrations.

Section

1

Surgical Anatomy Related to Cataract Surgery

THE VARIOUS LAYERS OF THE LENS

- Anterior and posterior capsule with subcapsular epithelium
- Cortex
- Epinucleus
- Nucleus

To study all the layers a good slit-lamp biomicroscopy has to be done with a well dilated pupil. This helps us to assess the type of cataract and to grade the hardness of the nucleus.

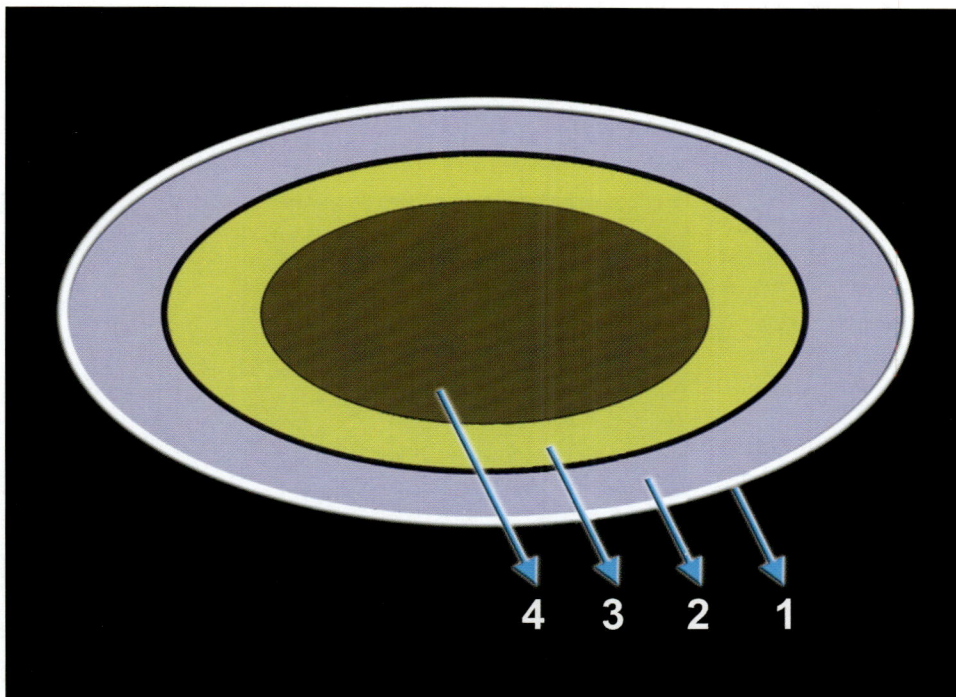

Fig. 1.1: Layers of the Lens—1-capsule, 2-cortex, 3-epinucleus, 4-nucleus

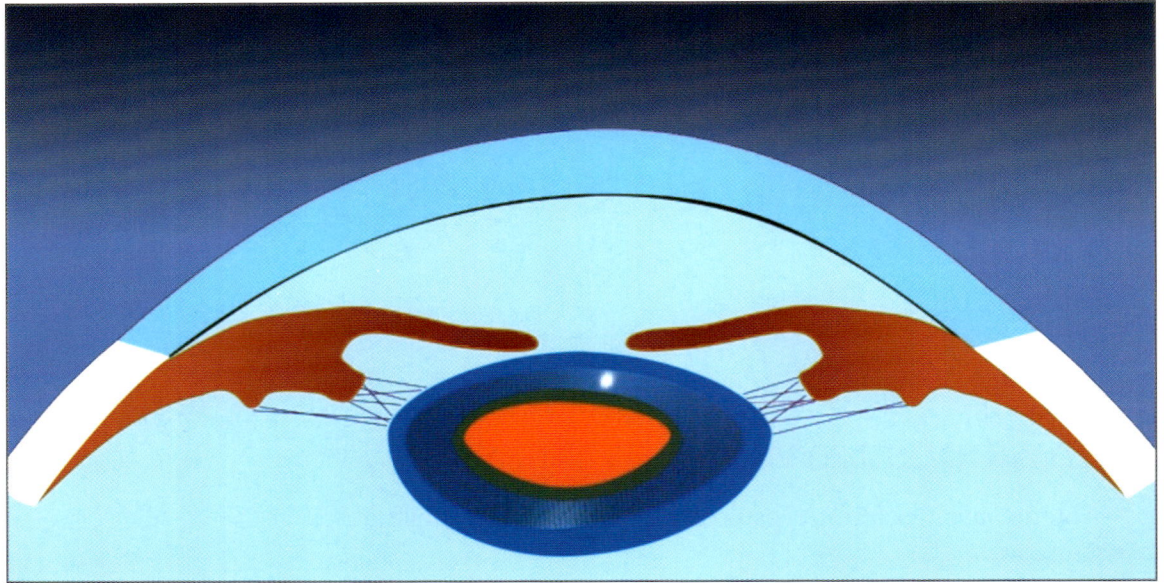

Fig. 1. 2: Peripheral corneas

Cornea

The peripheral corneal and limbal anatomy has to be understood before going into the surgical procedure
- Anterior limbus is the attachment of conjunctiva and Tenon's to the cornea
- Mid limbus is behind the blue line. It is important as the Descemets ends there
- Posterior limbus lies 1mm behind the mid limbus
- Care should be taken to prevent damage to the Descemets membrane while making the internal incision. The incision should be either anterior or posterior to its insertion. After making incision care should be taken while introducing the instruments into the eye. Phacotip and IOLs should not cause detachment of the Descemets membrane while introducing into the anterior chamber. Internal incision should be at least 1mm in the clear cornea to create a good valvular effect.

Corneal endothelium

Specular microscopy–normal count should be 1000 to 3500 cells/cubic mm. If cell count falls below 500/cubic mm, post-operative corneal edema occurs. Endothelium has no capacity to regenerate hence it is important to minimize damage to the endothelial cells during surgical maneuvers.

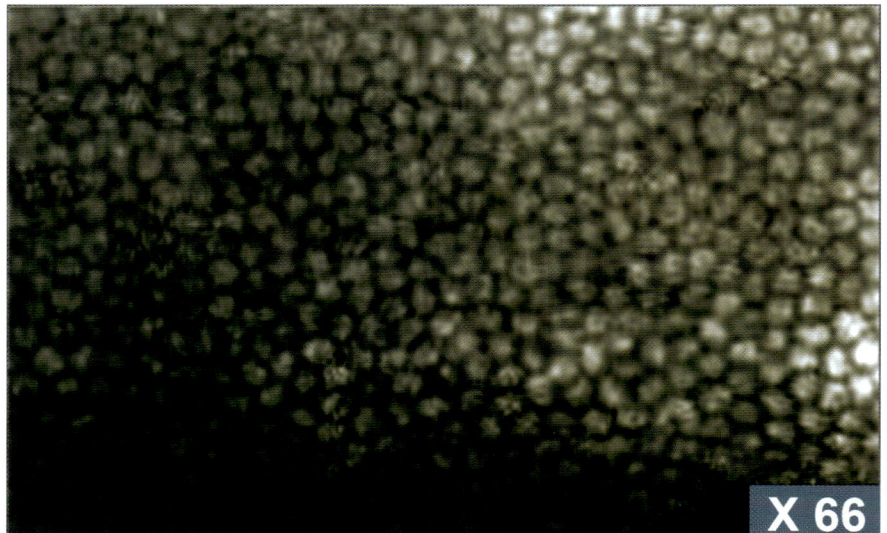

Fig. 1.3: Specular microscopic picture of normal corneal endothelium. Cells are similar in size and shape

2

Operating Room Setup

The operation room should be set up properly with well positioned air filters, sterilization units and the necessary aseptic measures have to be strictly followed to have a good outcome of the surgery. The surgeon should know thoroughly the functions of an operating microscope and should set it up well before starting the surgery.

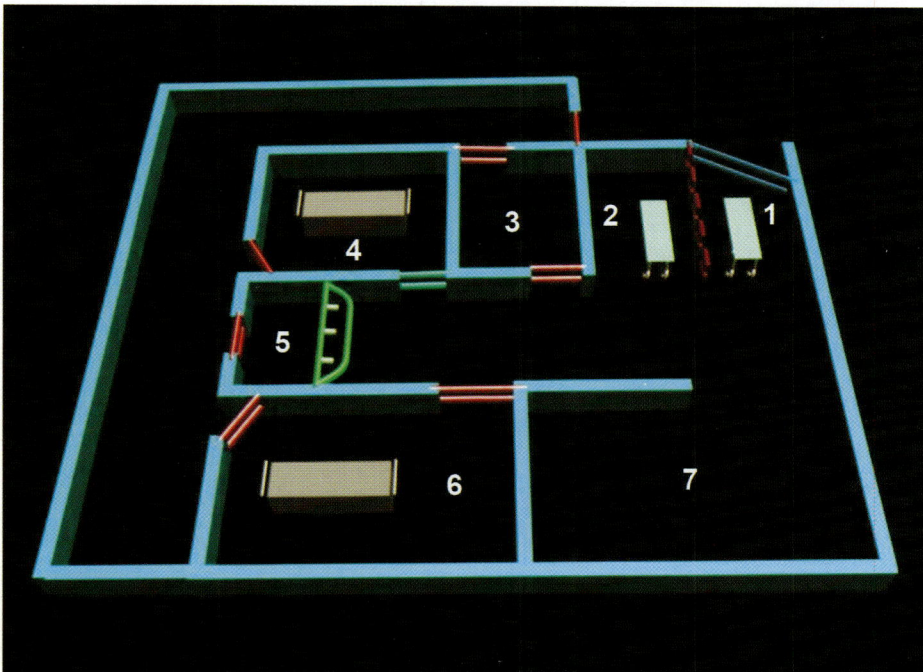

Fig. 2.1: OR set up (1) ward trolley (2) OR trolley (3) changing room (4) OR1 (5) wash area (6) Operating Room 2 (7) post-operative room

Air filters: The air in the operating room should be well filtered, as most of the bacteria and fungi are of diameter of 0.5 to 5 microns. High Efficiency Particulate Air filter system (HEPA) should be used. The system has a pore diameter of 0.3 microns and filters most of the bacteria and fungi. The filtered air is delivered by unidirectional laminar flow system kept over the operating table.

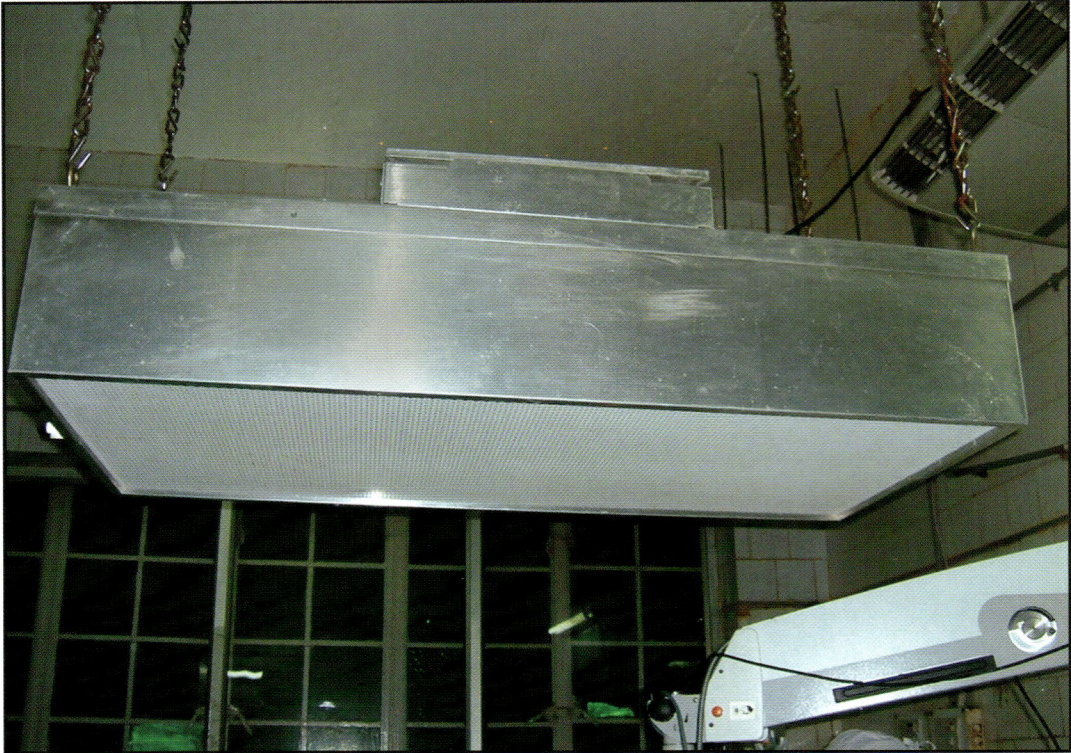

Fig. 2.2: HEPA (High efficiency particulate air filter) Cleaning and disinfection of OR

1. The OR should be washed thoroughly with soap and water.
2. The floor and two meters of OR walls should be washed with phenolic compounds.
3. The tables, chairs and stools in the OR should be wiped with 70% alcohol.
4. Formaldehyde fumigation–500 ml of 40% formaldehyde for every 1000 cu ft of space is used and it is kept closed for 8 to 10 hours.

Sterilization of Instruments

Dry heat: Used for sterilization of sharp instruments. Should be heated at 160° C for one hour 180° C for 20 minutes.

Autoclave: It is suitable for metallic ophthalmic instruments, linen, plastic and rubber items. Sharp instruments should not be autoclaved as they loose their sharpness.

They should be kept at 120° C and 15 psi pressure for 15 minutes

Flash sterilization: Done for emergency purposes. It is performed at 134° C and 34 psi pressure for 3 minutes for metal instruments and 10 minutes for linen, plastic and rubber items.

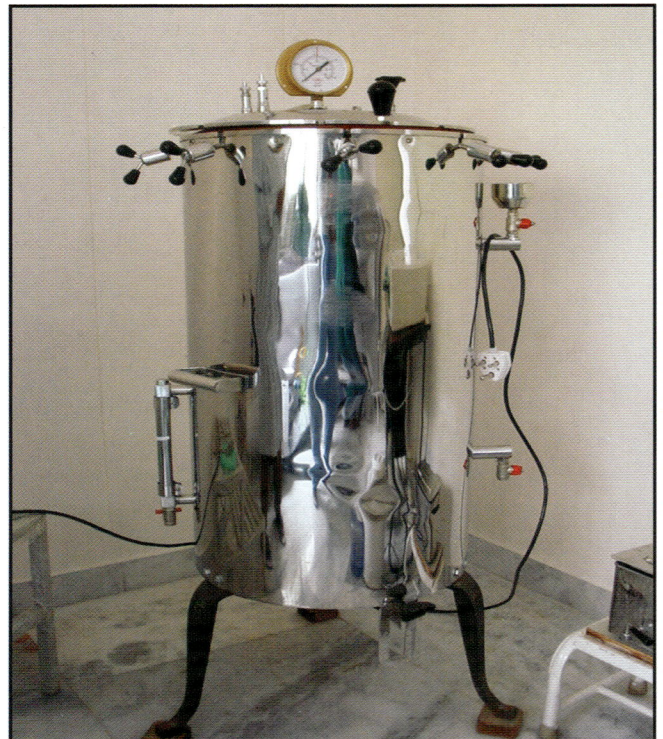

Fig. 2.3: Autoclave

Recently for fast and rapid sterilization cassette type of autoclaves (STATIM) are being used.

Filtration: This method is used for sterilizing irrigating fluids, intraocular air and gas injection.

Filtration is done using micropore filters having a pore diameter of 0.22 microns.

Chemical sterilization

2% Glutaraldehyde (Cidex)— used for sterilization of instruments which cannot be autoclaved as, sharp instruments, instruments made with plastic and rubber. The instruments should be soaked in

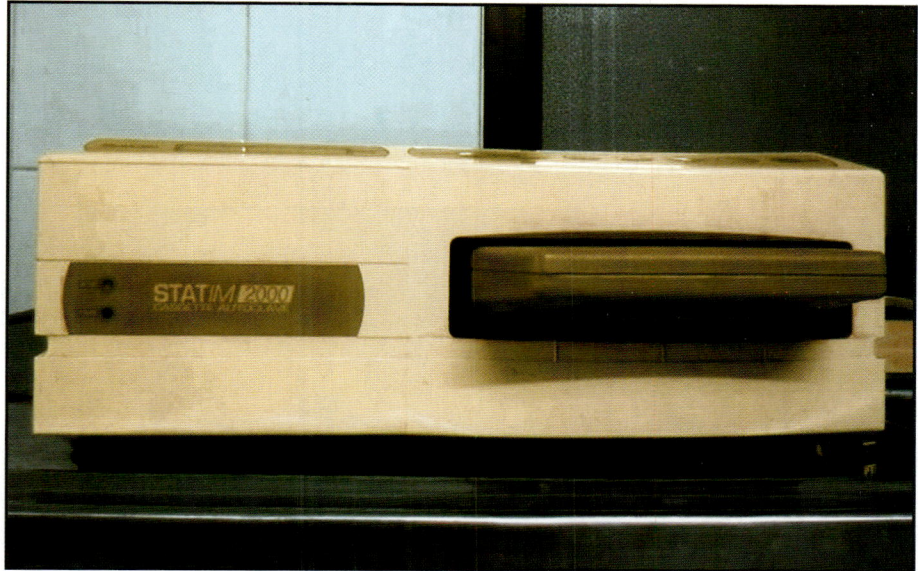

Fig. 2.4: Cassette autoclave (STATIM)

the solution for 3 hours. The instruments should be thoroughly washed with sterile normal saline or Ringer lactate before use.

Ethylene oxide (ETO)—ETO gas is used. It is effective and safe for sterilization of rubber tubes, vitrectomy cutters, sharp instruments, laser probes, cryoprobes, diathermy leads, etc. The minimum concentration required is 400 to 1000 mg / liter of space.

Operating table: Ideally one should have a motorized operating table with foot switch control.

Surgeon chair: It should also have motorized mechanism with hand rest for good control of hand movements.

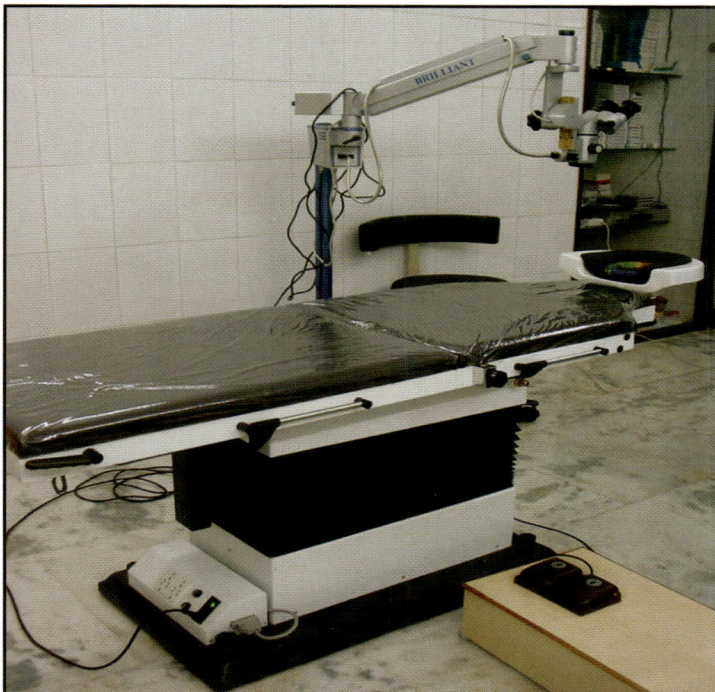

Fig. 2.5: Motorized operating table for adjustment of height

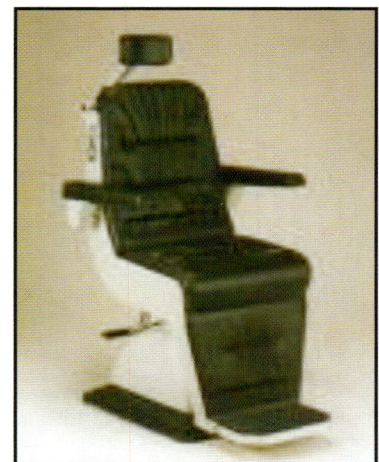

Fig. 2.6: Surgeon's chair— convenient height can be adjusted

OPERATING MICROSCOPE

Adjustments

Step 1:   Adjustment of eye pieces for refractive error

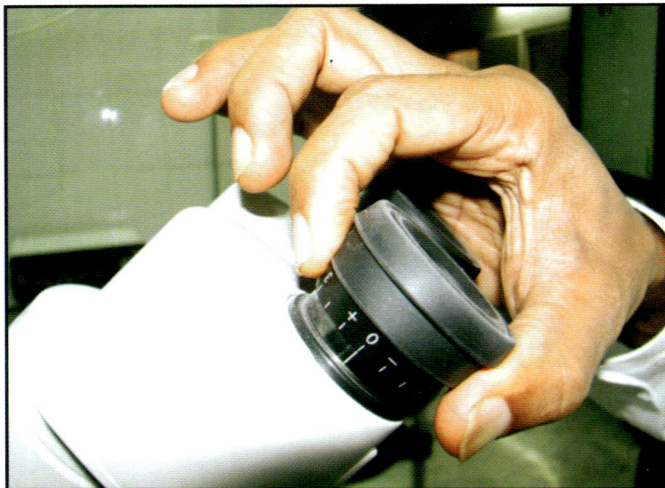

Fig. 2.7A: Adjustment of eye piece

Step 2:   Adjustment of Interpupillary Distance (IPD)

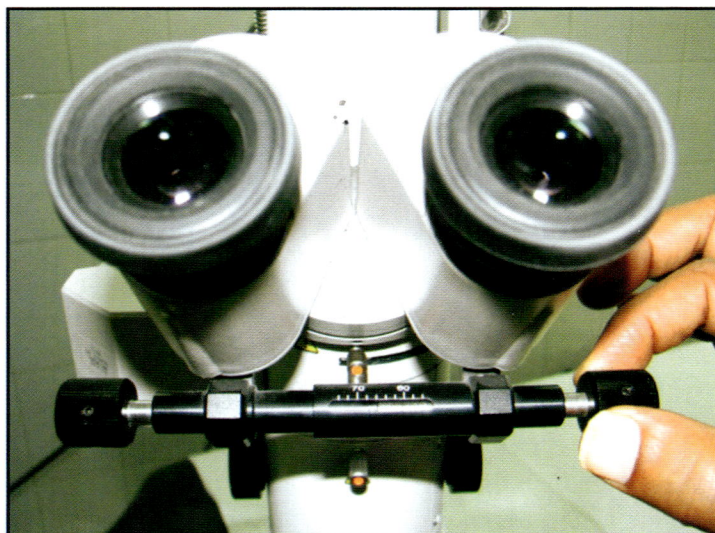

Fig. 2.7B: Adjustment of IPD

Step 3: Adjustment of rheostat for proper illumination

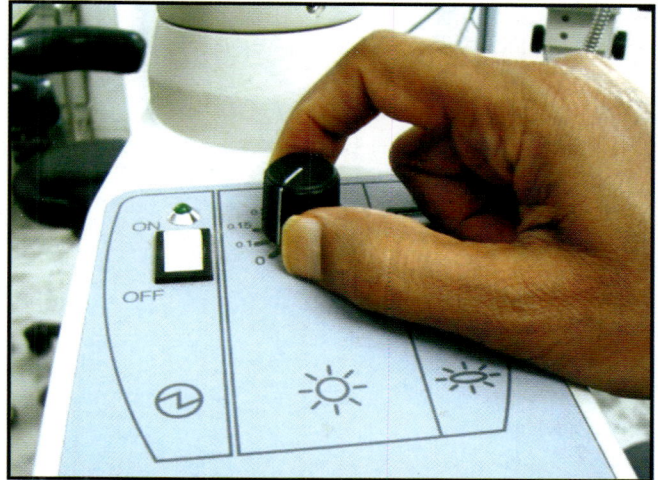

Fig. 2.7C: Adjustment of illumination

Step 4: Focusing

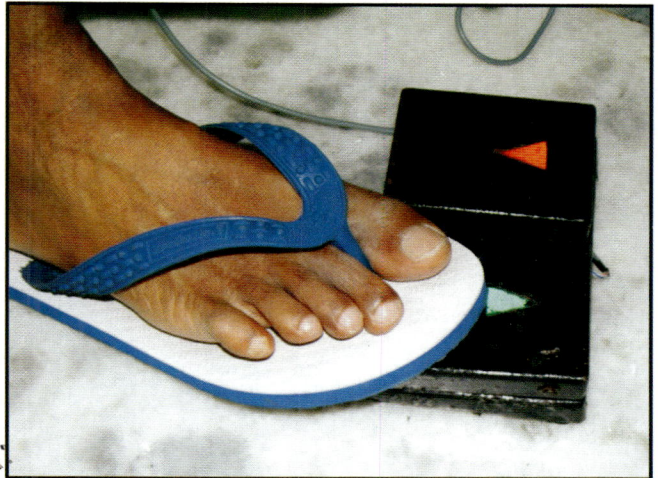

Fig. 2.7D: Focusing

Step 5: Adjustment of magnification

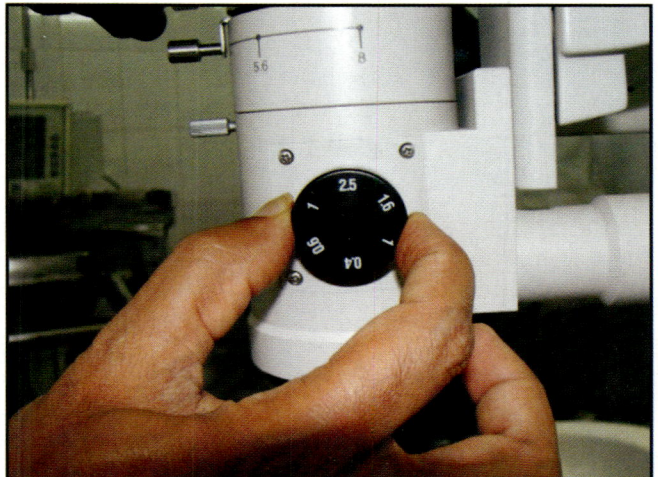

Fig. 2.7E: Adjustment of magnification

3

Preoperative Evaluation

AIM

- To determine if surgery is indicated or not
- To determine the visual prognosis following surgery
- To avoid intraoperative and post-operative complications.

HISTORY

- Visual loss—gradual or sudden
- Unilateral or bilateral
- Previous vision in BE
- Visual status in fellow eye
- Congenital cataracts—maternal history
- Redness of the eye
- Previous ocular surgery—cornea, glaucoma or retina
- Hypertension
- Diabetes
- Ischemic heart diseases
- Asthma
- Drug allergies
- Drug Usage - Corticosteroids
  - Antiglaucoma drugs
  - Anticoagulants
- Skin diseases
- Respiratory system
- CNS
- Mental health
- Rheumatoid arthritis.

SYSTEMIC EXAMINATION

A. Blood Pressure Recording

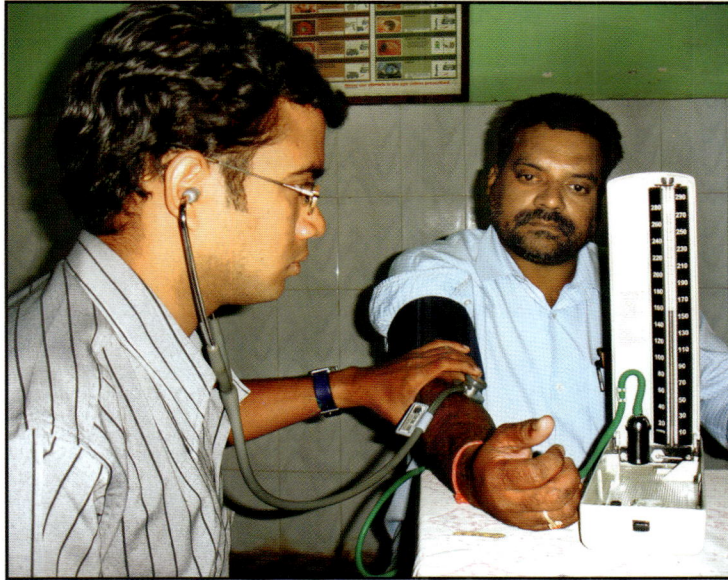

Fig. 3.1: Blood pressure recording

Blood pressure should be kept under control before taking up surgery. If the patient is a known hypertensive on treatment it is advisable to take ECG and Echo and take the opinion of a cardiologist as silent infarcts of the heart and brain is not uncommon.

If patient is on any anticoagulant therapy, it is advisable to discontinue it one week prior to surgery with the opinion of cardiologist.

B. Blood Sugar Estimation

It should be done routinely for all patients. A random blood sample should be examined. For all patients with history of diabetes a fasting blood sample and post lunch sample should be examined. For all these patients a single reading is not sufficient.

Glycosylated hemoglobin estimation is preferable in long standing diabetics.

Consent

An informed written consent from all patients or parents should be taken before the surgery. High-risk consent if necessary should be taken.

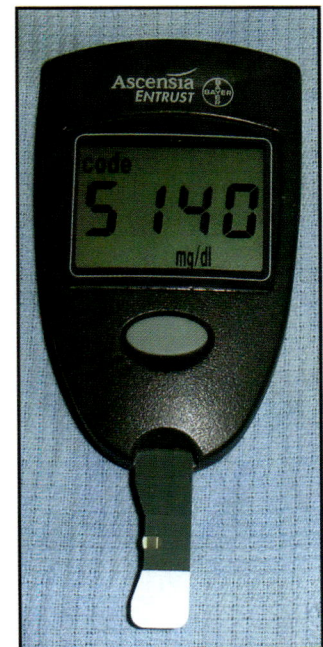

Fig. 3.2: Glucometer for bed side blood sugar estimation

4

Ocular Examination

Slit-lamp Biomicroscopy—Stage I (without dilatation) examine the

- Lids: Blepharitis, meibomitis, hordeolum, chalazion
- Conjunctiva: Palpebral, bulbar and fornices
- Cornea: Opacities, keratic precipitates, vascularization
- Anterior chamber: Depth (central and peripheral)
- Iris: Nodules, atrophic patches, synechiae, rubeosis
- Gonioscopy to visualize angle of the anterior chamber. It is advisable to do YAG PI if there is suspicion of occludable angle as preoperative dilatation for cataract surgery will result in acute attack of glaucoma.
- Pupil: Size, shape and reaction should be noted to plan for surgery
  - A miotic pupil should be ruled out
  - A sluggish reaction and no reaction should arouse the suspicion of fundus pathology and glaucoma.

Slit Lamp Biomicroscopy—Stage II (With dilatation) to examine the lens

Adjustments of slit-lamp

- Diffuse illumination
- Optical section
- Retroillumination
- The angle of illumination along the edge of the pupil
- Height of the beam reduced to size of the pupil

Note: The following points regarding the lens

- Type of cataract—cortical / nuclear, capsular / subcapsular
- Grading the density of cataract
- Intactness of zonule and capsule

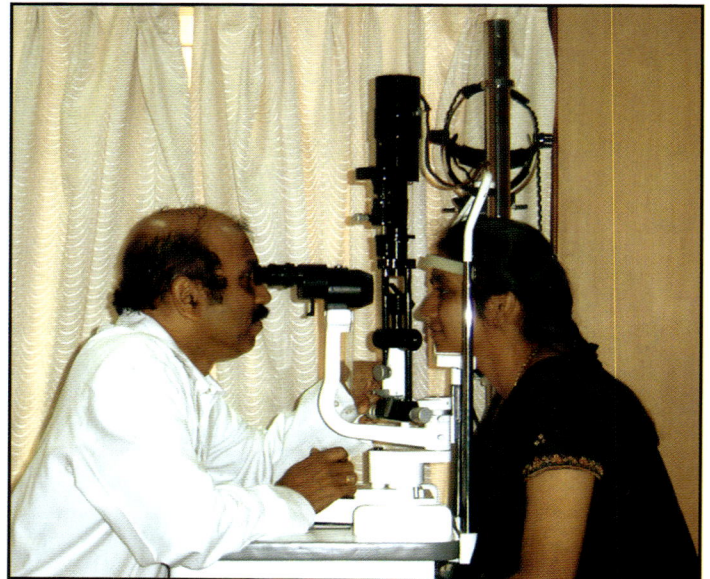

Fig. 4.1: Slit-lamp examination of anterior and posterior segments

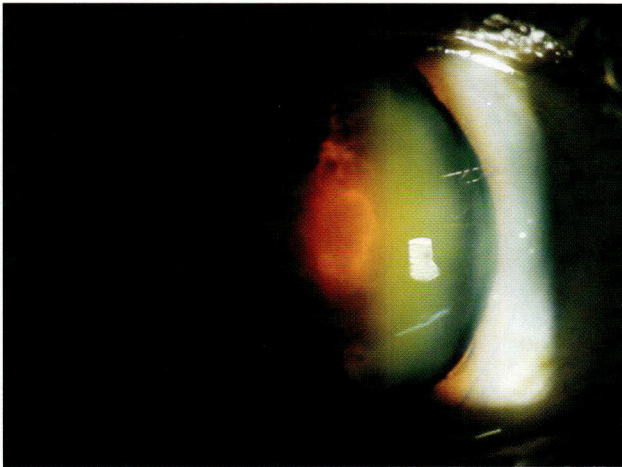

Fig. 4.2: Posterior polar cataract

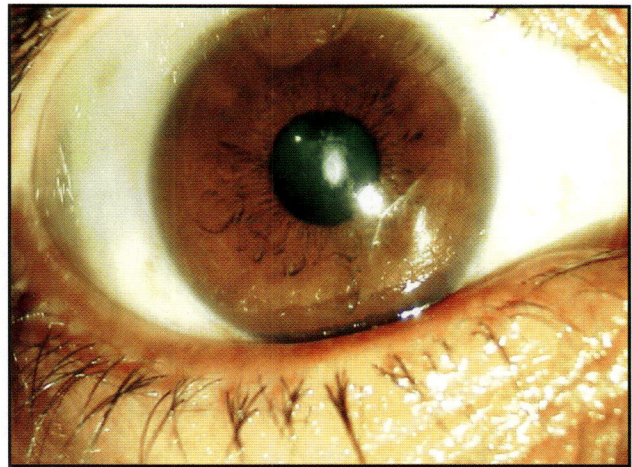

Fig. 4.3: Anterior polar cataract

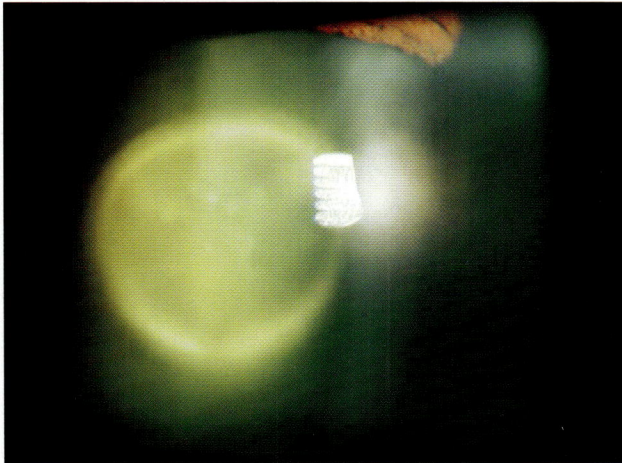

Fig. 4.4: Zonular cataract

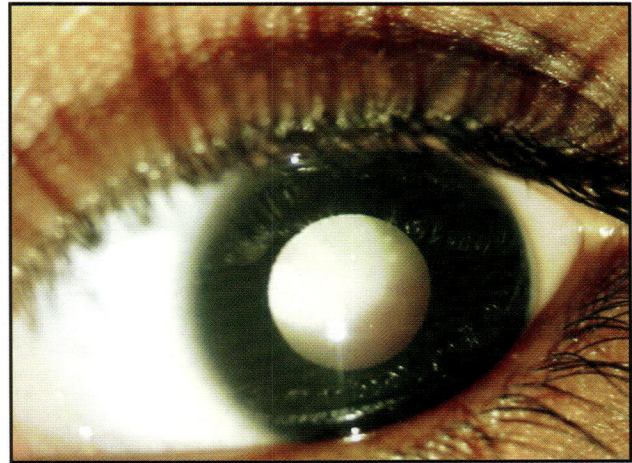

Fig. 4.5: Senile cataract

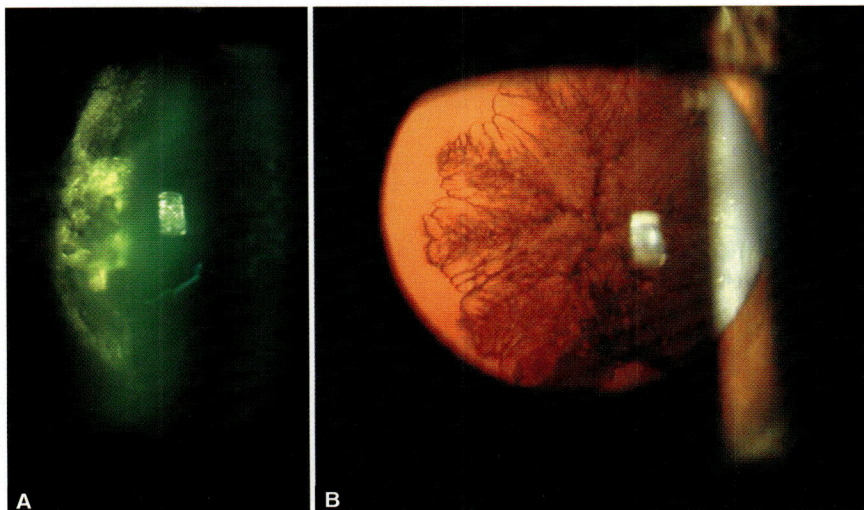

Figs 4.6A and B: Posterior subcapsular cataract

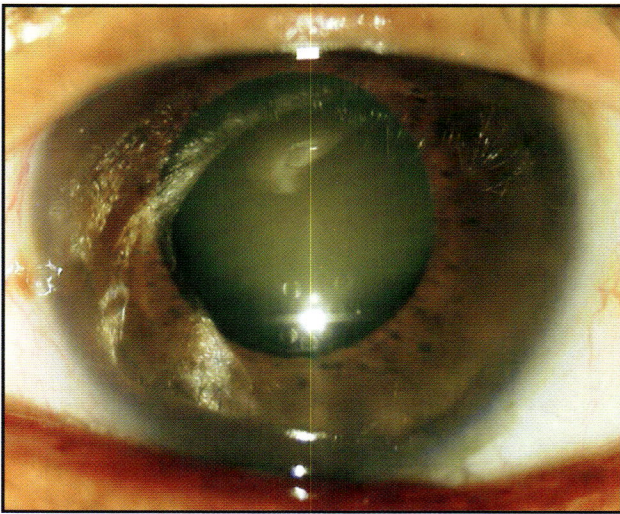

Fig. 4.7: Nuclear cataract

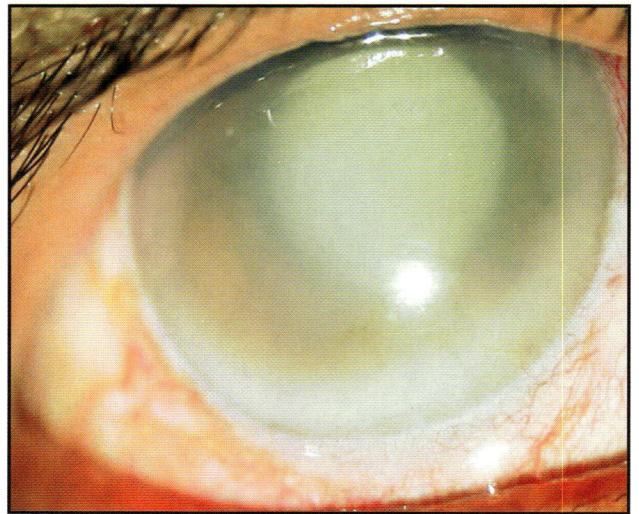

Fig. 4.8: Hypermature cataract (secondary glaucoma)

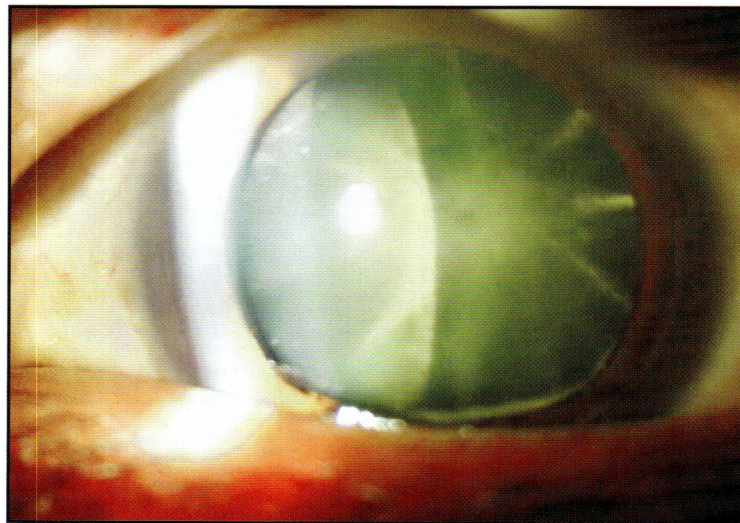

Fig. 4.9: Traumatic cataract

Grading of Cataract

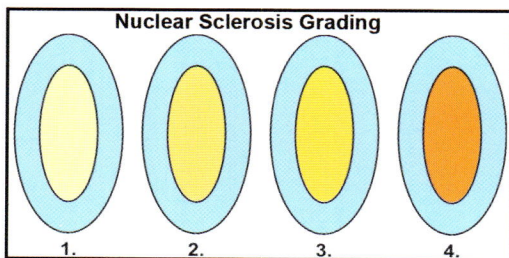

Fig. 4.10: Grading of nucleus for estimation of hardness

Table 4.1: Grading of cataract

Grade	Color
1/2	Slight-Yellowing
1	Definite-Yellowing
2	Very-deep-Yellow
3	Yellow-Organge
4	Orange-Brown

POSTERIOR SEGMENT EXAMINATION

- Direct ophthalmoscopy
- Indirect ophthalmoscopy
- Slit-lamp biomicroscopy with +78 D lens
- When there is a dense cataract it is advisable to take Ultrasound B-scan to exclude retinal detachment and vitreous hemorrhage.

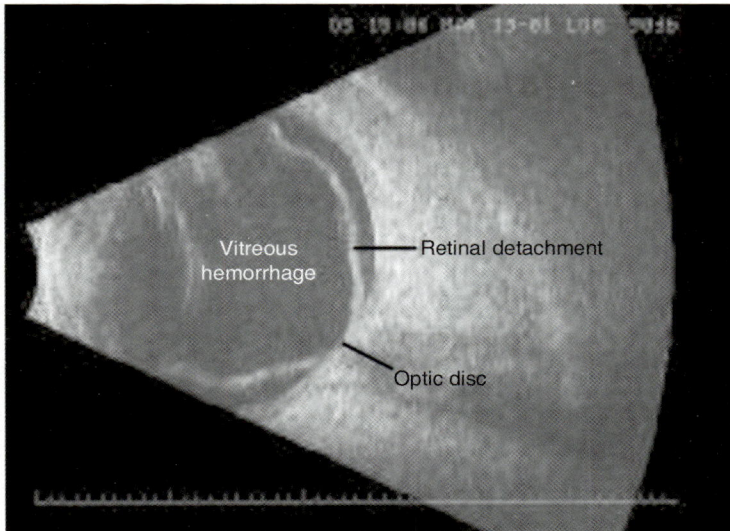

Fig. 4.11: Ultasound B-scan in a case of mature cataract showing RD

In cases where there is sluggish pupil and RAPD and degenerative diseases of retina like retinitis pigmentosa and optic atrophy, it is advisable to do electrophysiological test to predict the post-operative results. The commonly done tests are—

- ERG
- EOG
- VEP

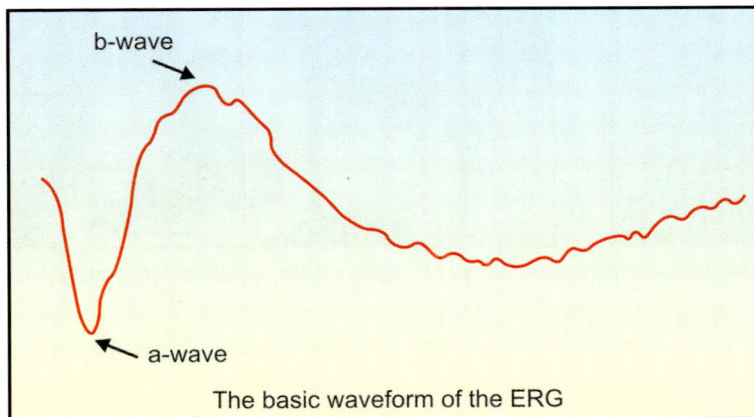

Fig. 4.12A: Normal ERG to assess retinal function in dense cataracts

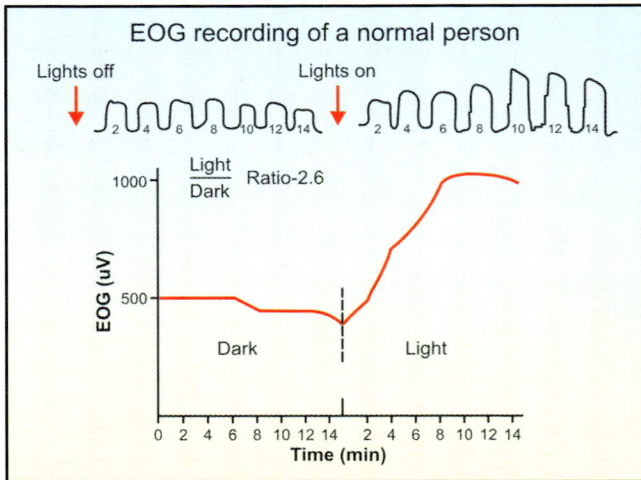

Fig. 4.12B: Normal EOG to assess retinal function

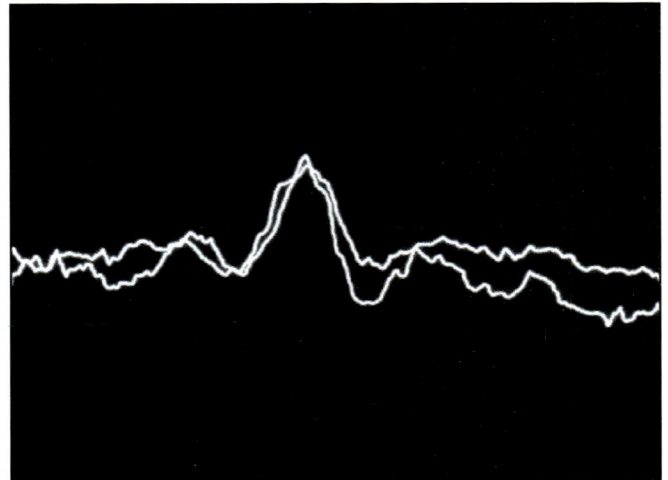

Fig. 4.12C: VEP to evaluate optic nerve function in dense cataract RE normal pattern LE sub normal pattern

Intraocular Pressure

It is ideal to record IOP with applanation tonometer if available. Schitz tonometer may record false readings in some of the conditions as in

- Myopia previous ocular surgery
- Glaucoma suspects
- Cataract associated with glaucoma
- Patients on antiglaucoma therapy

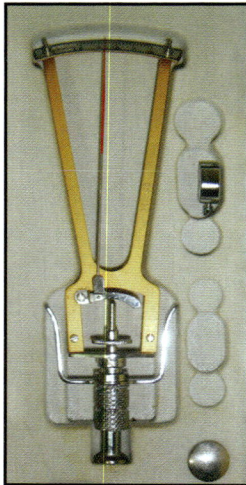

Fig. 4.13A: Schiotz tonometer

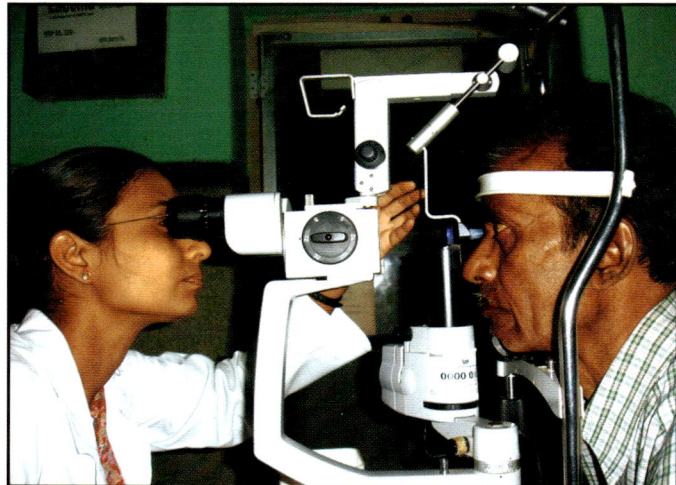

Fig. 4.13B: Applanation tonometry

Patency of nasolacrimal duct—it is tested by

- Regurgitation test under slit-lamp
- Dye test using mercurochrome
- Syringing test

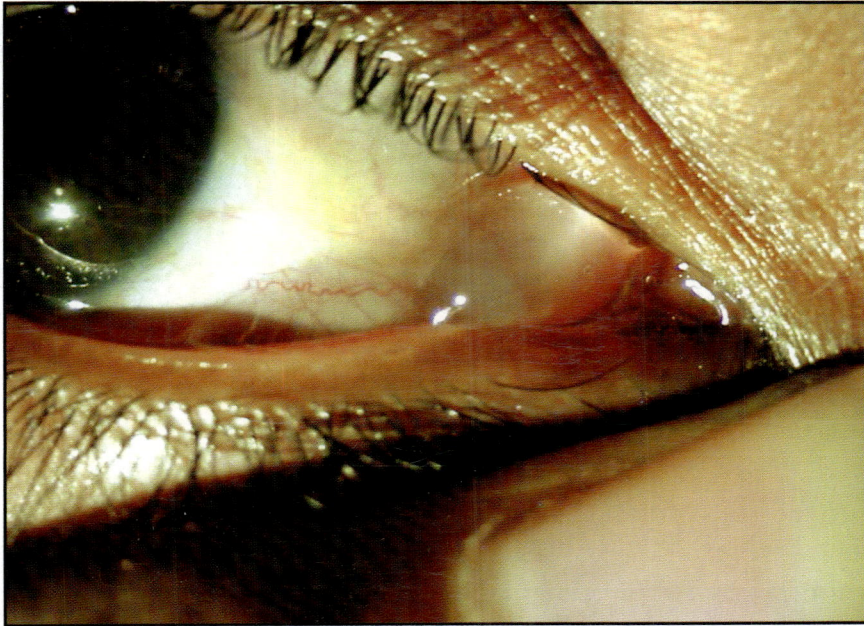

Fig. 4.14: Regurgitation test under slit-lamp pressure is applied and regurgitation of fluid is seen

Specular microscopy

Corneal endothelial study is indicated in cataract associated with corneal degenerations, dystrophies, post trauma, post-surgical and post-keratoplasty.

Normal endothelial count 1000 to 3500 cells / cu mm. Any thing less than 500 / cu mm will result in corneal edema. In cases with a compromised endothelium it is advisable to use a high molecular weight viscoelastic (see chapter 8) during surgery.

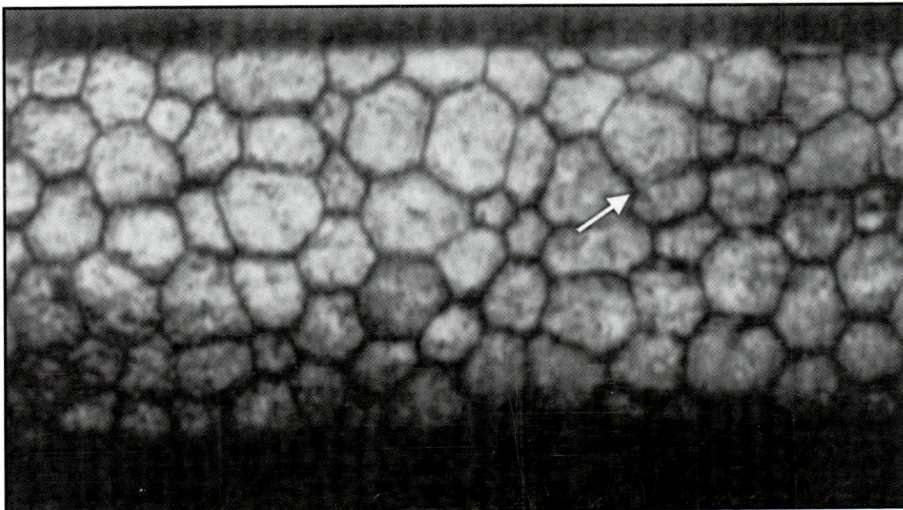

Fig. 4.15: Specular microscopy of abnormal endothelium cells are showing pleomorphism and polymegathism

5

Biometry

Biometry is done by—

Keratometry: • To get an idea of preoperative astigmatism and its axis
• To measure corneal curvatures (horizontal and vertical)
• To diagnose keratoconus

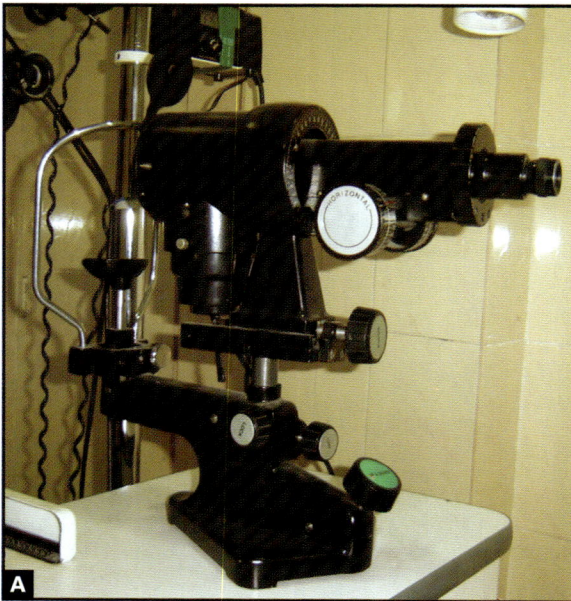

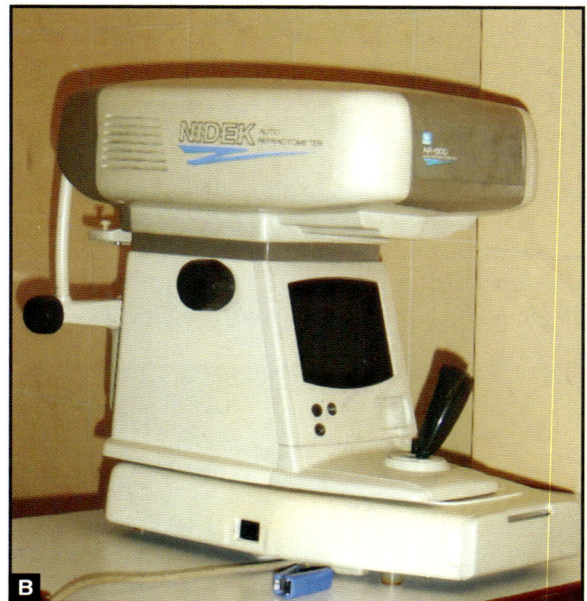

Figs 5.1A and B: Keratometry manual and automated

• When to repeat Keratometry?
• K-reading more than 47D or less than 40D
• Previous keratorefractive surgery
• Difference of more than 1D between the two eyes
• Dense cataract where the patient is not able to fix properly
• Corneal diameter less than 11 mm.

A. Scan Ultrasonography

• Contact method (easy to do)
• Immersion method (accurate)

Optical Coherence (IOL Master) (More accurate)

When to repeat A-scan?

Axial length less than 22 mm or more than 25 mm.

In high myopes with posterior staphyloma.

Difference in axial length between both the eyes more than 0.33 mm.

When you are planning for multifocal IOL and refractive lens surgery, it is preferable to do A-scan of the other eye also and calculate the IOL power.

IOL Master

The principle is optical laser coherence interferometry. It is a non contact method. It is 5 times more accurate than contact A-scan.

It takes K-reading and axial length including AC depth simultaneously and thus saves time.

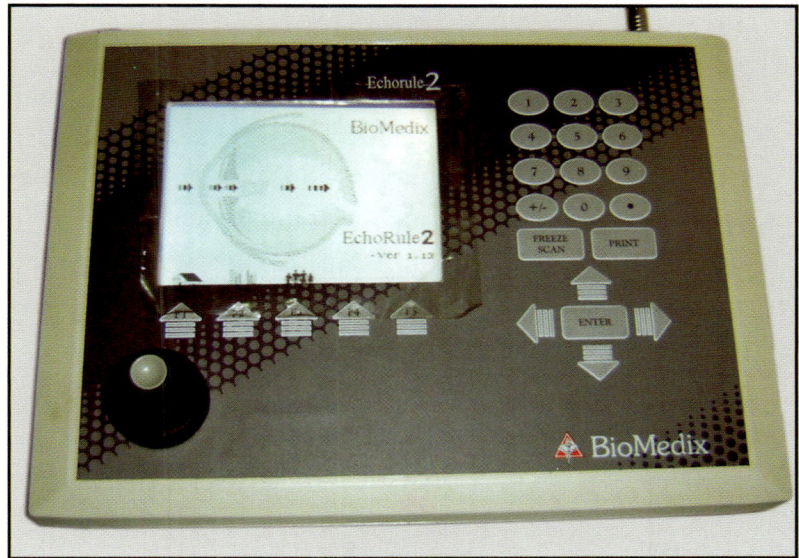

Fig.5.2: A-scan

Disadvantages: High cost of the equipment. Cannot be used in dense cataract (Laser coherence interferometry)

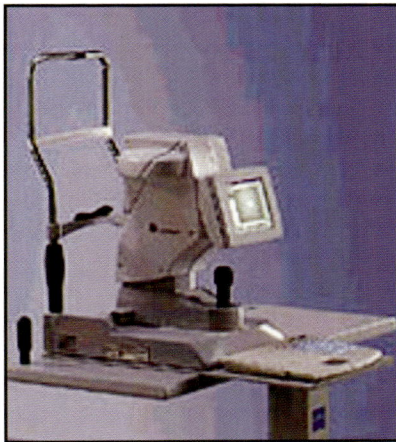

Fig. 5.3A: IOL master (courtesy ziess)

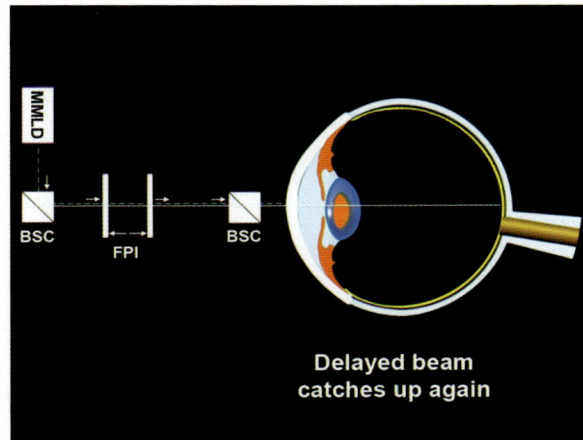

Fig. 5.3B: Principle of IOL master

IOL Power Calculation is Difficult in

- Pediatric cataracts
- Previous corneal refractive surgery
- Eyes with silicone oil.

IOL Power Calculation

SRK I (Sanders, Retzlaff and Kraff) Formula:
$$P = A - 2.5L - 0.9K$$

SRK ll Formula:
>   For too long and short eyes
> $P = A - 2.5L - 0.9K + C$

C = SRK11 correction factor for long and short eyes
AL 21 to 22 mm add 1D
AL 20 to 21 mm add 2 D
AL 10 to 20 mm add 3D
AL more than 24.5 mm subtract 0.5 D

Third Generation Formulae

Key to highly accurate IOL power calculation is being able to predict D (ELP)—effective lens placement for any given patient and IOL
>   SRK/T – uses a constant
>   Holladay I– uses surgeon's factor
>   Holladay II– uses AC depth
>   Hoffer Q formula– AC depth

IOL POWER IN DIFFICULT SITUATIONS

In children

>   Depending on age:
>   If less than 2 years — Using biometry, calculate the IOL power as usual and under correct by 20%.
>   In children between 2 and 8 years. Under correct the IOL power by 10%.
>   Using axial length:
>   17 mm - 25 D
>   18 mm - 24 D
>   19 mm - 23 D
>   20 mm - 21 D
>   21 mm - 19 D

Post-Refractive Surgery

1. *Calculation method:*
   - Three parameters must be known. K readings, preoperative (refractive surgery) refraction and post-operative (refractive surgery) refraction.
   - The change in refraction at corneal plane is calculated, i.e. Preoperative refraction–Postoperative refraction.
   - This is subtracted from original K readings (prerefractive) to obtain present K reading
     Present K = mean preoperative K– Change in refraction.

2. *Trial hard contact lens method:*

   A hard Planocontact lens with a known base curve is used. Normal refraction is done. Refraction with hard contact lens in place is done. When both these refractions are equal, the base curve of the contact lens is the K reading of cornea.

3. *Corneal topography:*

   It detects any defects on the anterior and posterior surfaces of the cornea accurately as in early keratoconus, postrefractive surgeries.

Post-vitreoretinal Surgery

1. *Silicone oil:*

   It acts as a negative lens in the eye. Silicone oil filled eyes record a high axial length on A-scan as the refractive index of silicon oil is less than that of vitreous. Ultrasound waves travel slowly, i.e. 980 m/sec compared to normal vitreous 1532 m/sec this gives a high axial length measurement. To get the correct axial length.
   Velocity in silicone oil 980 m/sec

   $$\text{Actual AL} = \text{Measured AL} \times \frac{\text{Velocity in silicone oil}}{\text{Velocity in vitreous}} = \frac{980}{1532} = \text{AL} \times 0.63$$

2. *Scleral buckle:*

   Causes myopic shift. So IOL of lesser power is required.

6

Anesthesia

Cataract surgery is usually done under local anesthesia, but nowadays with the advent of phacoemulsification, it is being done even under topical anesthesia. General anesthesia for cataract surgery is reserved only for few special cases.

Local Anesthesia

Orbital nerve block

- Retrobulbar
- Peribulbar
- Facial
- Parabulbar
- Topical

Drugs used in local anesthesia—

Short acting—1% procaine, 1% chloroprocaine
Intermediate acting—2% lidocaine (xylocaine), 2% mepivacaine
Long acting—0.5% bupivacaine, tetracaine

Orbital block

Commonly used drugs for orbital block 2% xylocaine + 0.5% bupivacaine + epinephrine 1:20000 + hyaluronidase.

Epinephrine prolongs the duration of anesthesia due to vasoconstrictor effect. It is contraindicated in patients with hypertension and cardiovascular problems.

Hyaluronidase allows rapid diffusion of anesthetic by hydrolysing the hyaluronic acid in the extracellular spaces 7.5 to 15 units /ml of anesthetic solution should be added.

Retrobulbar block: 23 G needle is introduced into the orbit through the lower lid between the medial two-thirds and lateral one third into the muscle cone (intraconal). Needle tip should always be directed towards the eyeball. 3 to 5 ml of anesthetic is injected slowly.

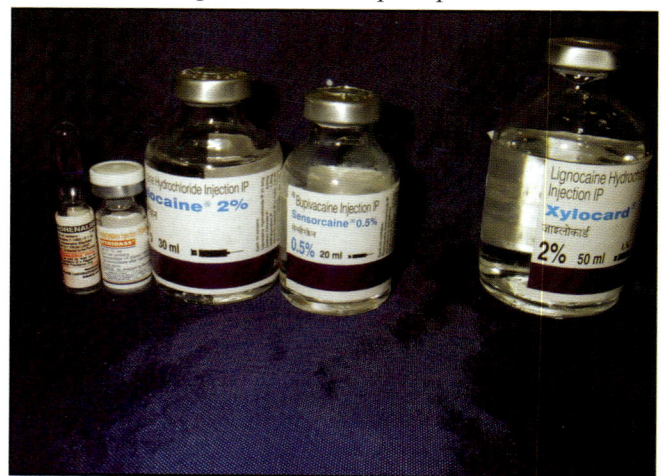

Fig. 6.1: Local anesthetic drugs

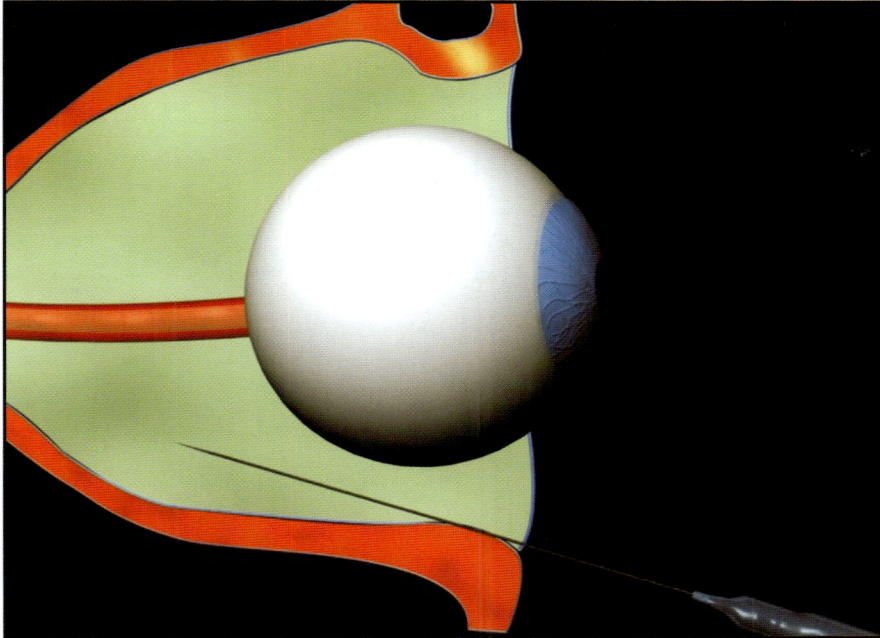

Fig. 6.2A: Retrobulbar block

Peribulbar block: In this method the anesthetic is injected extracoronally. 7 to 10 ml of anesthetic is taken. 4 to 5 ml is injected inferotemporally by passing the needle through the lower lid at the same point as in retrobulbar block. If necessary 2 to 3 ml is injected superonasally through the upper lid.

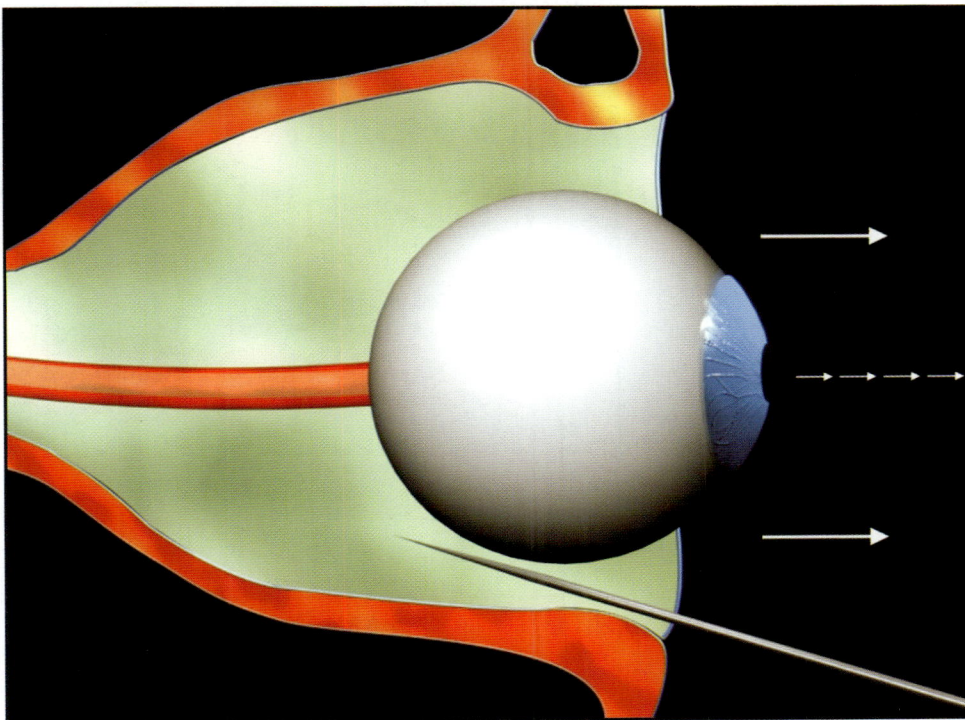

Fig. 6.2B: Peribulbar block

Parabulbar block: In this method the anesthetic is injected into the subtenon's space after making an opening in the conjunctival and tenons 2 to 3 mm from the limbus. The injection is given with a special cannula which is about 10 mm in length and allows entry into the posterior tenon's space. Injection is usually given in the superonasal quadrant. 1 to 1.5 ml of solution is injected.

Facial block: It is infrequently used, but sometimes it may be required to block the facial nerve to avoid sqeezing of the lids by contraction of orbicularis oculi muscle. The nerve may be blocked at various points along its course.

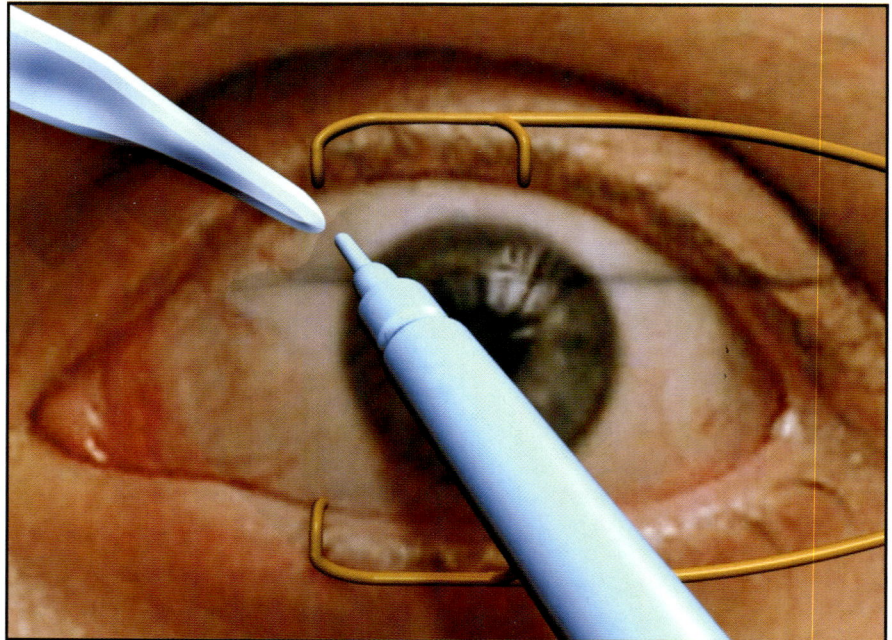
Fig. 6.2C: Parabulbar block local anesthetic is injected underneath the tenon's capsule

- External canthus—Van lint's technique
- Zygomatic arch—Atkinson's technique
- Condyle of mandible—O'Brien's technique
- Stylomastoid foramen—Nadbath's technique.

To achieve good preoperative hypotony, a super pinkie is applied over the closed eyeball over an eye pad for about 10 to 15 minutes. In the absence of pinkie intermittent pressure with a palm may be applied.

Complications

- Retrobulbar hemorrhage
- Optic nerve damage
- Anaphylaxis
- CNS depression
- Needle perforation of globe

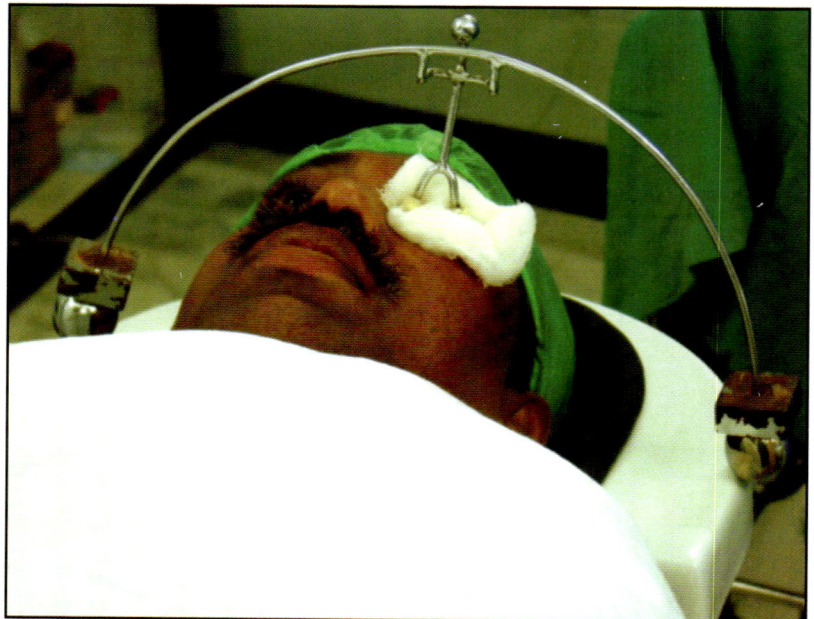
Fig. 6.3: Super pinkie placed after injection

Needle Perforation

Flow chart 6.1: Needle perforation of globe can occur

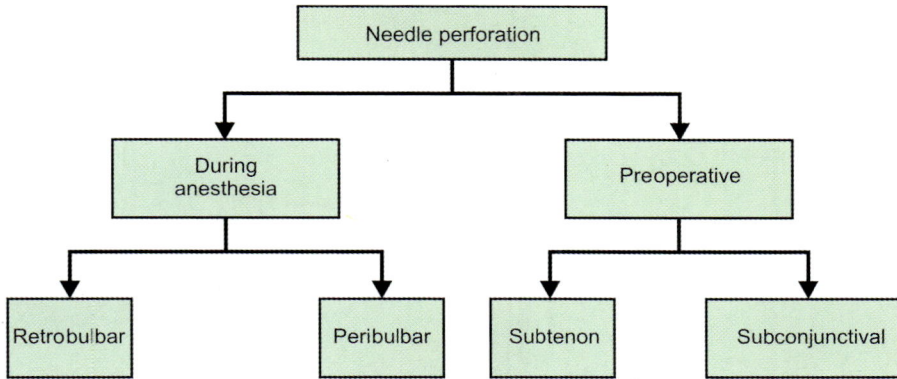

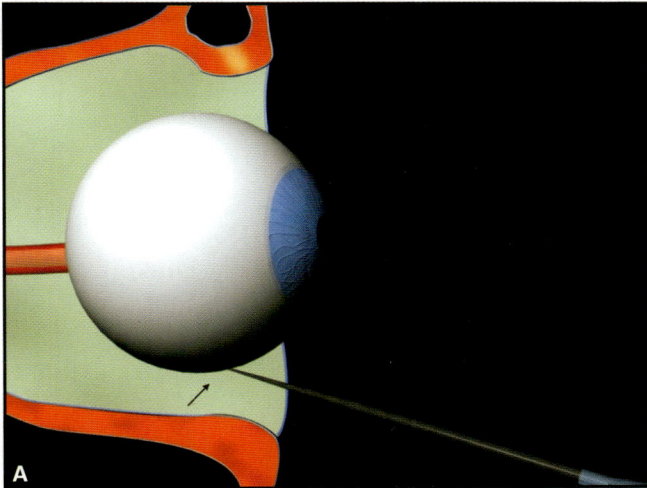

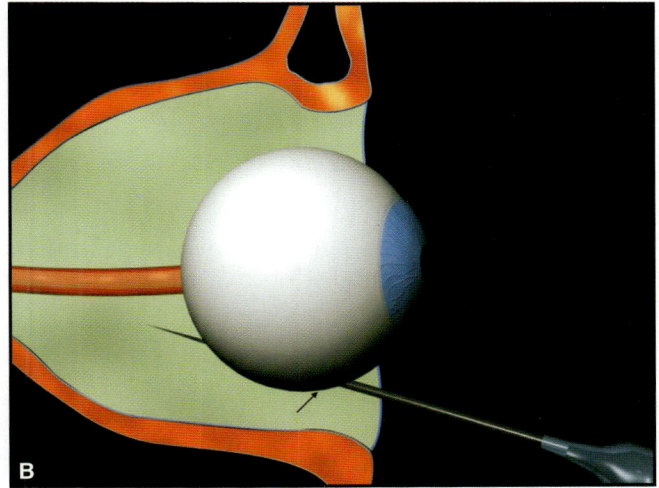

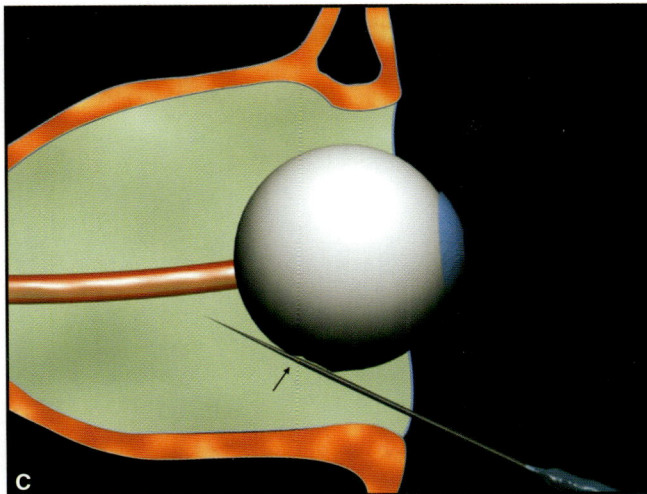

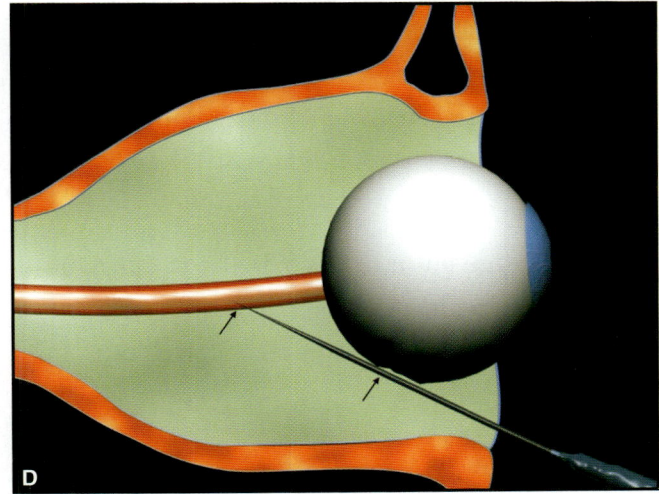

Needle perforation

During anesthesia

Preoperative

Retrobulbar

Peribulbar

Subtenon

Subconjunctival

Figs 6.4A to D: A. Needle penetration, B. Needle perforation, C. Laceration, D. Optic nerve

Predisposing factors

- Altered anatomy:
  1. Large globe > 26 mm
  2. Staphyloma
  3. Enophthalmos
  4. Post-RD buckle surgery
- Uncooperative patient.

Diagnosis

- Suspect in high-risk cases
- Severe pain
- Increase in IOP immediately followed by subsequent fall
- Corneal clouding
- Pupillary constriction
- Loss of red reflex
- Sudden discoloration under the conjunctiva
- Fundus examination to confirm perforation and to localize the lesion
- B-scan to look for vitreous hemorrhage and retinal detachment.
  Loss of vision is either due to vitreous hemorrhage, retinal-detachment or optic atrophy.

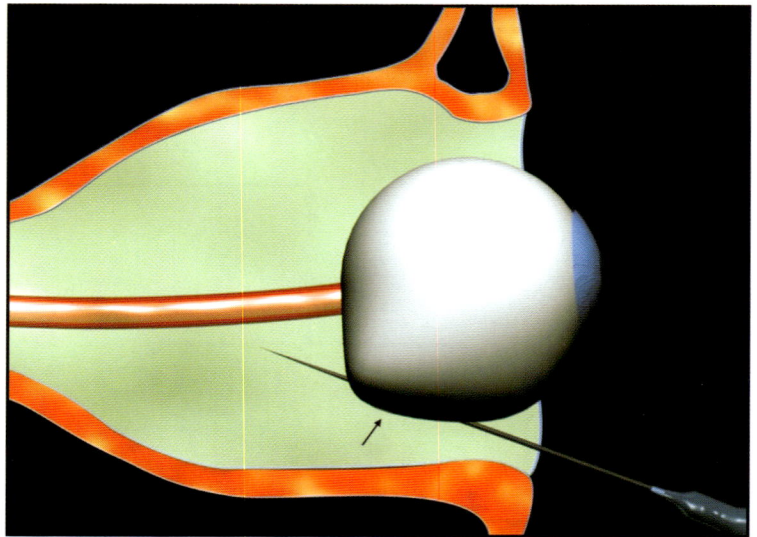

Fig. 6.5: Needle perforation of posterior staphyloma

Management

- Hypotony- Exploration and closure
- Vitreous hemorrhage- Vitrectomy
- Retinal detachment-Vitrectomy and scleral buckle
- Choroidal detachment-
  1. Small- Observe
  2. Large- Drain
- Retinal tear-LASER photocoagulation
- Proliferative vitreoretinopathy-Vitrectomy

Precautions

- Block is given in primary position, not with the patient looking upwards
- Enter at the level of the equator
- Do not change direction till 7 mm depth
- Check for resistance
- Check for corneal clouding
- High-risk cases need to be given modified topical/ subtenon's injection.

Topical

Drugs used - 1% preservative free xylocaine
0.5% proparacaine
0.5% to 1% tetracaine

It blocks the afferent nerves of the cornea and conjunctiva (long and short ciliary nerves, nasociliary nerves and lacrimal nerves).

Drops should be instilled 20 to 30 min before surgery and limited numbers of instillations are advised. Patient is asked to fix at the microscope light with both eyes open during surgery.

Intracameral (injection into anterior chamber) if necessary (if the patient complains of pain) is added. 1% preservative free xylocaine (xylocard) 0.1-0.2 ml may be given by doing a paracentesis.

General anesthesia—Indications for GA in cataract surgery are:
Pediatric patients
Mentally ill patients
Patients who are apprehensive
In patients with staphylomatous eyes where local blocks are contraindicated.

7

Surgical Procedure

SUPERIOR RECTUS SUTURE— FOR STABILIZING THE GLOBE

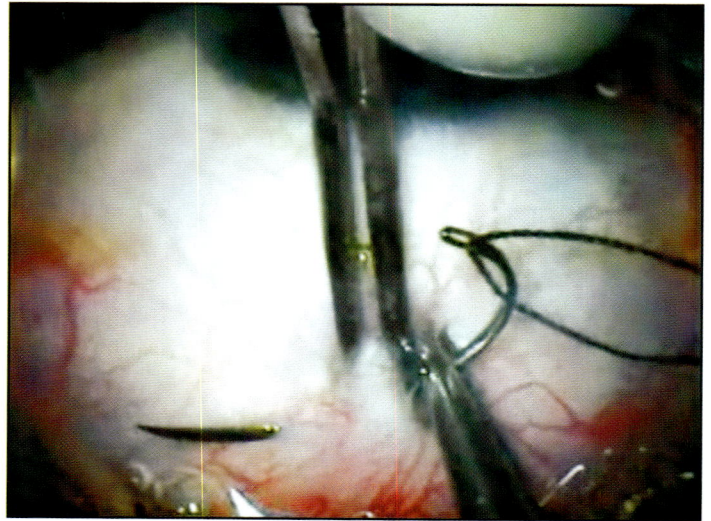

Fig. 7.1A: Superior rectus tendon suture

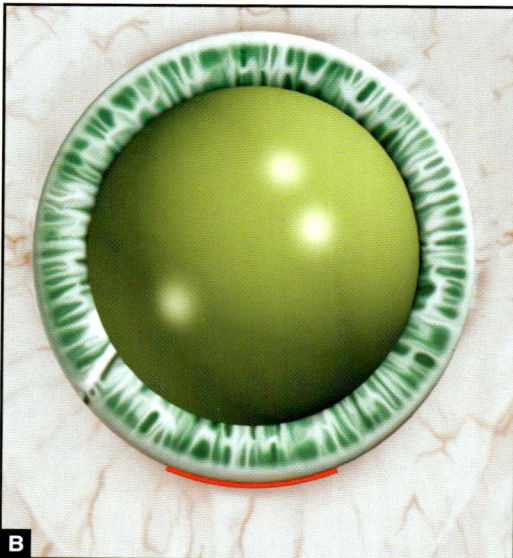

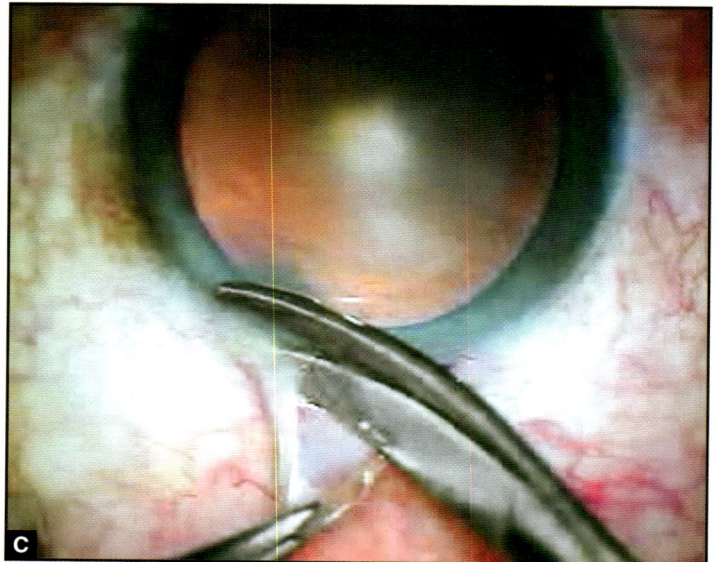

Figs 7.1B and C: Conjunctival incision

Conjunctival Incision

Made with a Westcott's scissors

- Incision made from 11 O' clock to 1 O' clock position close to the limbus (fornix based)
- Ideally made from one end to the other.
- Large opening is not advisable.

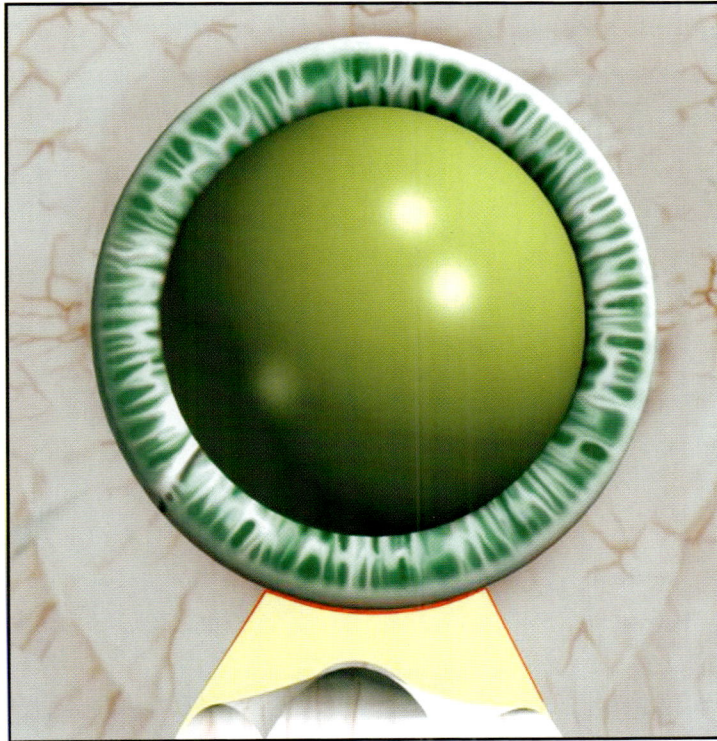

Fig. 7.1D: Conjunctival flap is reflected

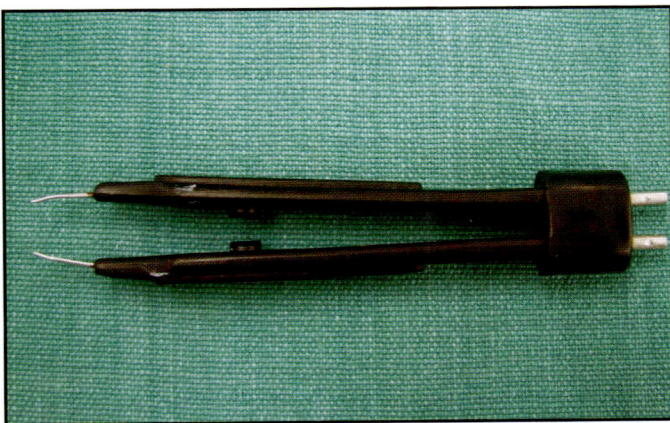

Fig. 7.2A: Bipolar cautery tip

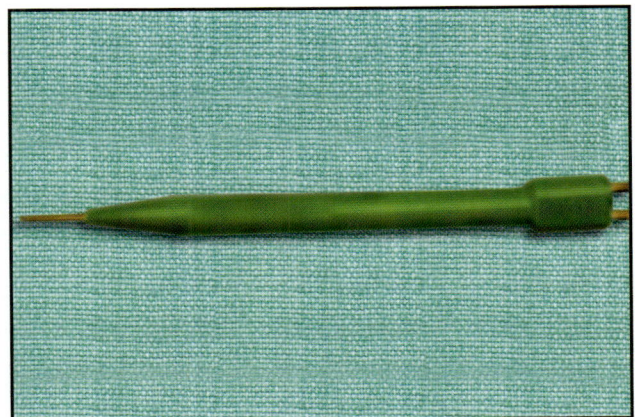

Fig. 7.2B: Eraser cautery tip

Cautery

- Bipolar cautery
- Eraser cautery or unipolar cautery
    - Bipolar wetfield cautery is preferable.
    - Unipolar eraser cautery if available is ideal as it causes
    - Minimal trauma to the tissues.

Heat cautery is not advisable as it may induce scleral necrosis and thinning

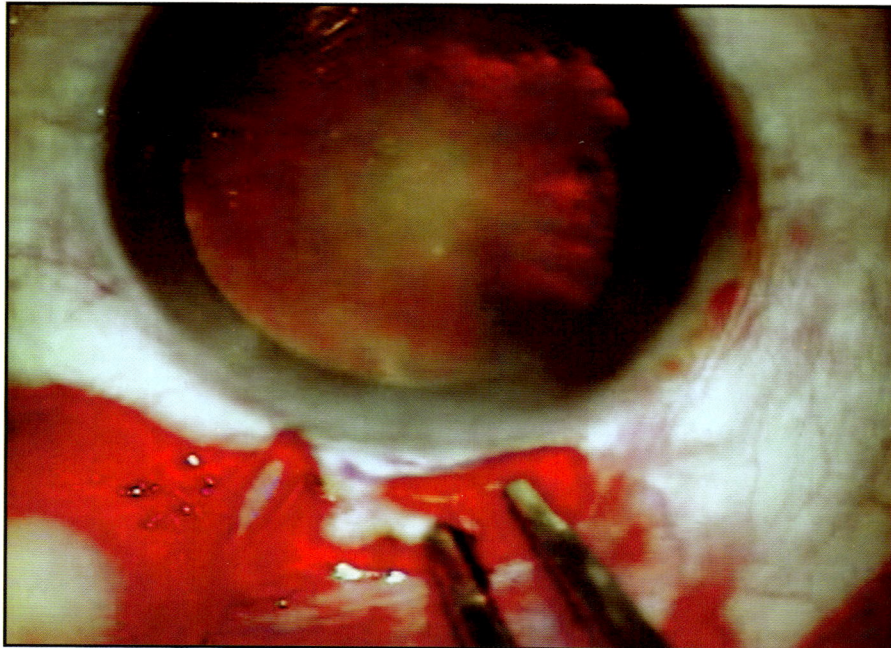

Fig. 7.2C: Bipolar cautery being used

Excessive cauterization may cause

- Scleral necrosis
- Scleral shrinkage
- High postoperative astigmatism
- Damage to the ciliary body causing postoperative uveitis
- Damage to the conjunctiva at the incision site
- Delayed wound healing.

Scleralcorneo Incisions

Ideal incision should be self sealing without sutures and should not induce any unwanted astigmatism.
Richard Kratz was the first scientist to create a scleral incision away from the limbus for cataract surgery.
Girard and Hoffman introduced the construction of a sclerocorneal tunnel.
Paul Ernest was the person to introduce the one way valve incision for self sealing wound.

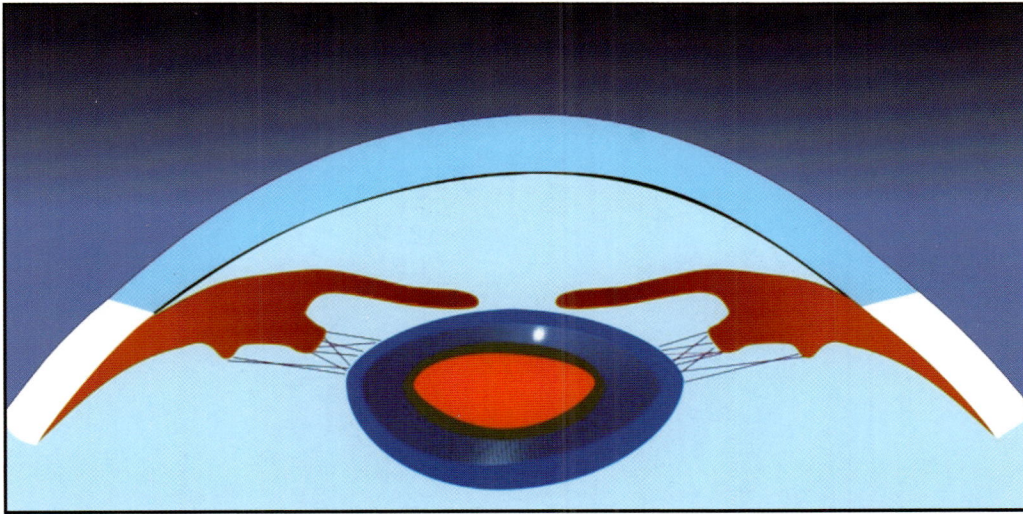

Fig. 7.3: Surgical limbus

It is very important that the operating surgeon be knowledgeable about the various aspects of different types of sclerocorneal incisions to avoid many intraoperative and postoperative complications

- Position of the incision
- Site of the incision
- Depth of the incision
- Width and length of the incision.

Position of the incision

Temporal Incision

Advantages

- Induces minimal astigmatism
- Easy access into anterior chamber as superior orbital rim does not come in the way
- Minimal effect of Bell's phenomenon when surgery is being done under topical anesthesia
- No pooling of fluid in the conjunctival sac.

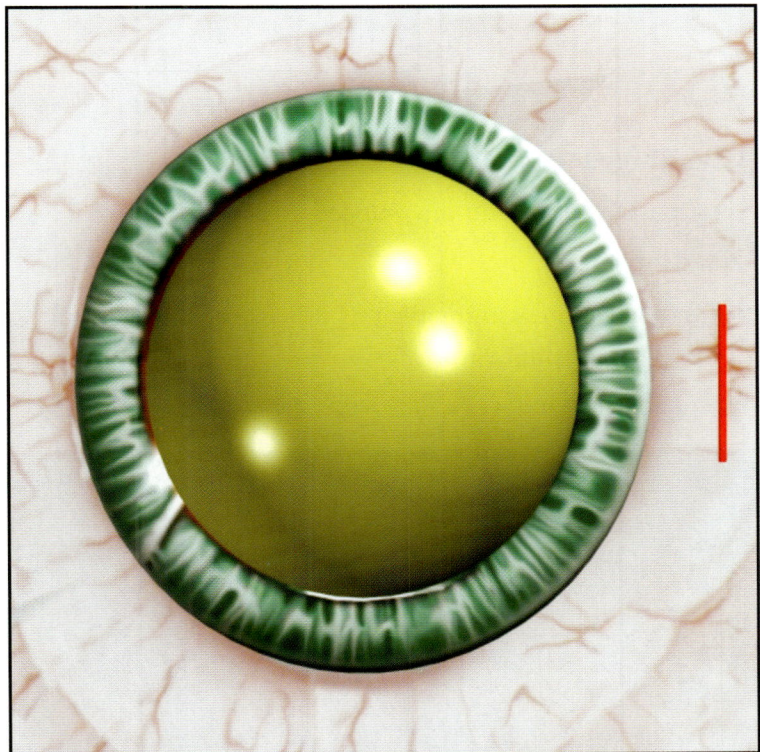

Fig. 7.4A: Temporal incision

Superior Incision: It is done by most of the surgeons.

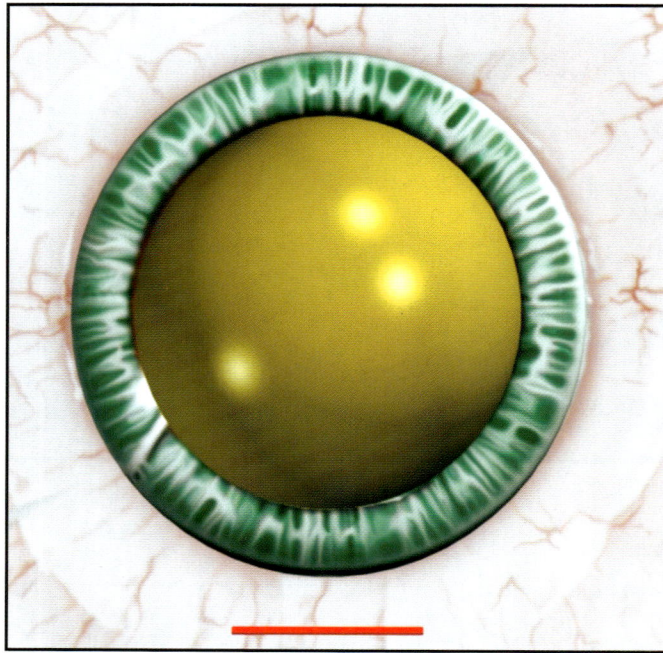

Fig. 7.4B: Superior incision

Advantages

- Operative scar and any subconjunctival hemorrhage will be hidden under the upper lid.

Disadvantages

- Induces more astigmatism as it is close to the visual axis
- Superior orbital rim comes in way during many operative maneuvers.

Incision corresponding to the steepest meridian

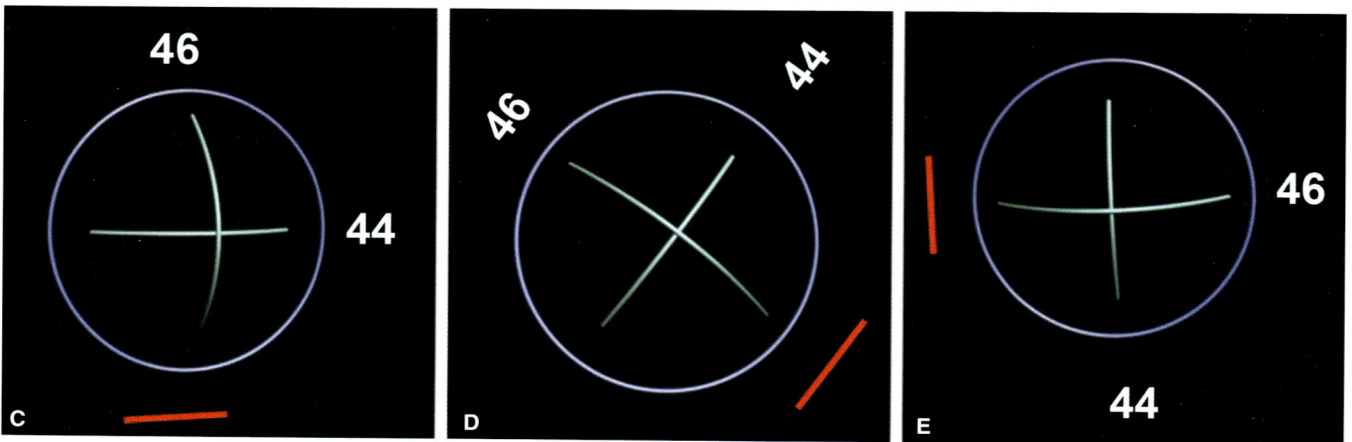

Figs 7.4C and E: Incision is taken along the steeper K meridian

Steepest meridian is marked by doing a preoperative keratometry. Incision is made along the greatest K value.

Site of the incision

Sclerocorneal tunnel incision

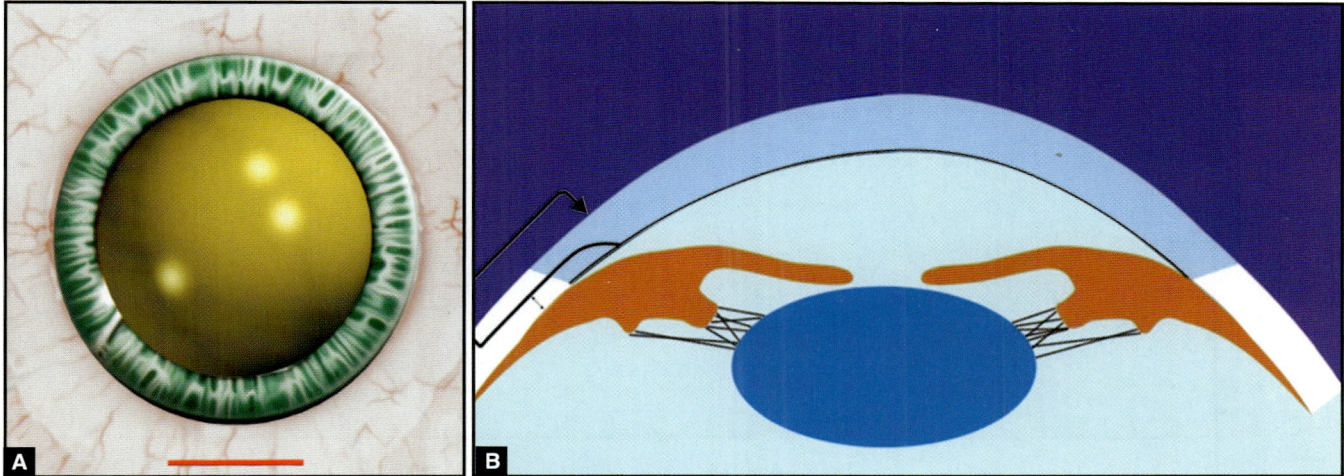

Figs 7.5A and B: Sclerocorneal incision

Advantages

1. Intraoperatively anterior chamber is well maintained and corneal endothelial damage is minimized.
2. IOP is kept under control and thus decreases the incidence of choroidal hemorrhage.
3. Surgery takes less time as there are no sutures to apply.
4. Postoperatively less scarring, less astigmatism and less inflammation compared to conventional ECCE incision.

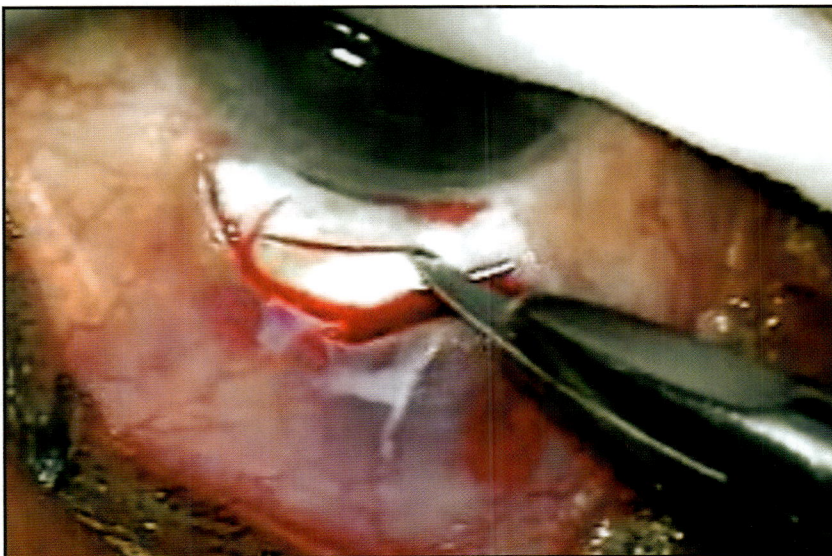

Fig. 7.5C: Sclerocorneal incision being marked

Clear Corneal Incision

Fine was the first person to introduce it.
Incision is made in the cornea anterior to the limbal vascular arcade.

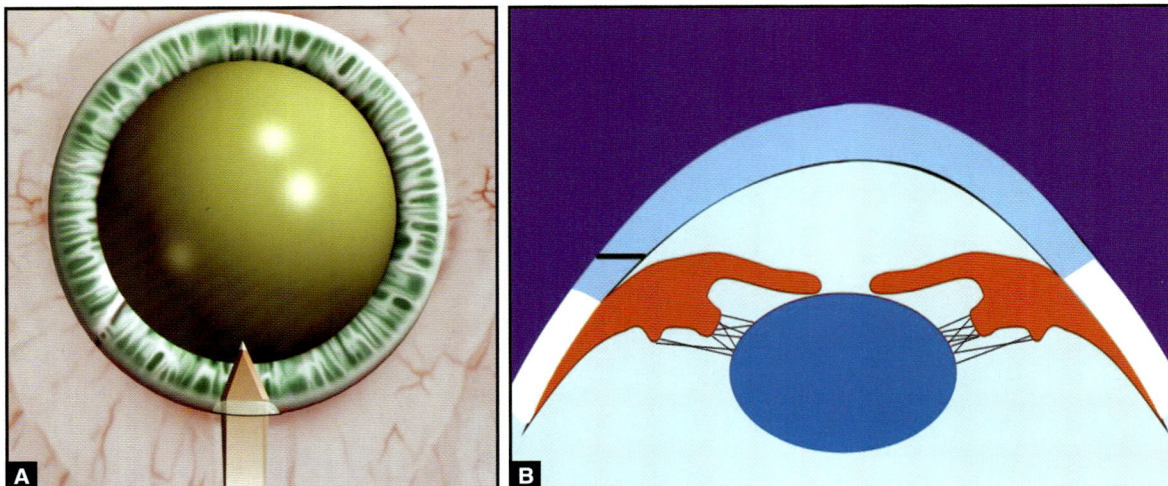

Figs 7.6A and B: Clear corneal incision

Advantages

- Surgery can be done under topical anesthesia
- Temporal incision can be easily made
- Minimal conjunctival scarring as conjunctiva is not cut
- Useful in cases of previous filtering surgery
- Less time and fewer instruments are needed.

Disadvantages

- Poor wound stability compared to scleral incision with increased risk of postoperative wound leak and infection.

Indications

- Wherever there is increased tendency of bleeding as in patients with anticoagulant therapy, with blood dyscrasias, diabetes and chronic alcoholism.

Contraindications

- Cases who have undergone radial keratotomy
- Peripheral corneal degenerations.

Near clear corneal incision

Situated 0.50 mm behind the vascular arcade

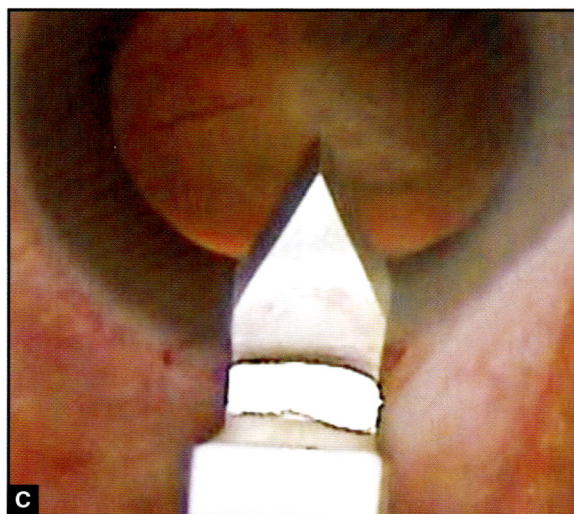

Fig. 7.6C: Clear corneal incision with a keratome

Advantages

- Has almost all advantages of corneal incision
- Induces relatively less astigmatism than corneal incision
- Healing will be fast due to closeness to the vascular arcade
- Good wound stability compared to corneal incision.

Disadvantages

- Ballooning of conjunctiva due to sub conjunctival passage of fluid during surgery leading to obscuration of surgical field.
- Increased incidence of subconjunctival hemorrhage.

Most of the present day surgeons do a clear corneal or near clear corneal incisions, this being an era of phacoemulsification and foldable IOLS.

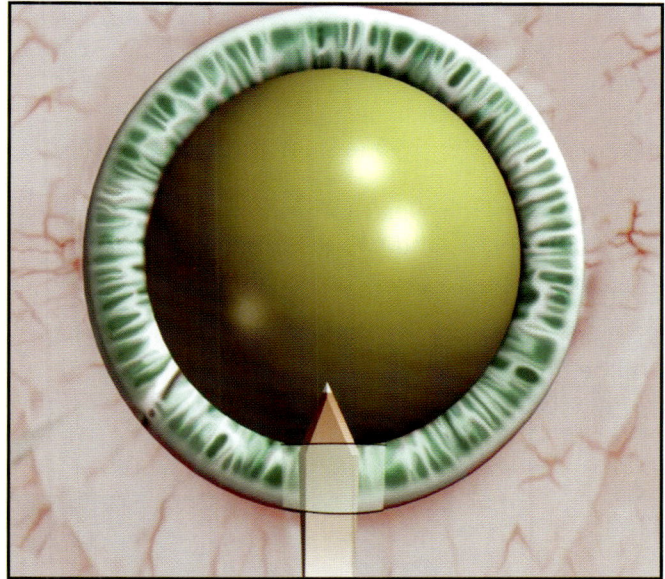

Fig. 7.6D: Near clear corneal incision

Size of Incision

It depends on the size of the nucleus to be delivered and the type of IOL to be placed.

For a rigid IOL the size of the incision should be about 6 mm.

For a foldable IOL 2.5 to 3.2 mm would suffice

Increase in the size of the incision causes an increase in the against the rule induced astigmatism

An incision of less than 3 mm will not cause any wound sag and hence no astigmatism.

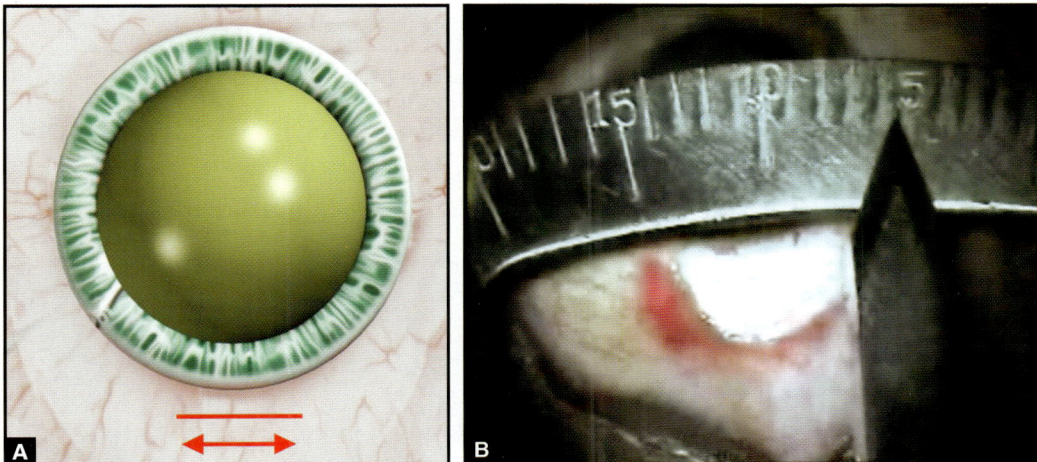

Figs 7.7A and B: Showing the length of incision in SICS measured with calipers

Depth of incision: In clear corneal and near clear corneal incision depth would be around 300 to 400 microns.

In sclerocorneal incisions, the depth is about 0.2 mm or 1/3 rd the thickness of the cornea (200-300 microns).

Thin flaps may lead to buttonholing of the flap and improper sealing of the wound.

Length of the tunnel

In clear corneal incision the width of the incision will be around 2 mm.

In sclerocorneal incisions it will be 2.5 to 3.5 mm wide.

Table 7.1: Shows the relationship between wound size and astigmatism

Incision length	Astigmatism against the rule (Dioptre)
3 mm	0
4 mm	1
5 mm	2
6 mm	3
7 mm	3.7
8 mm	4.5
9 mm	5.25
10 mm	6

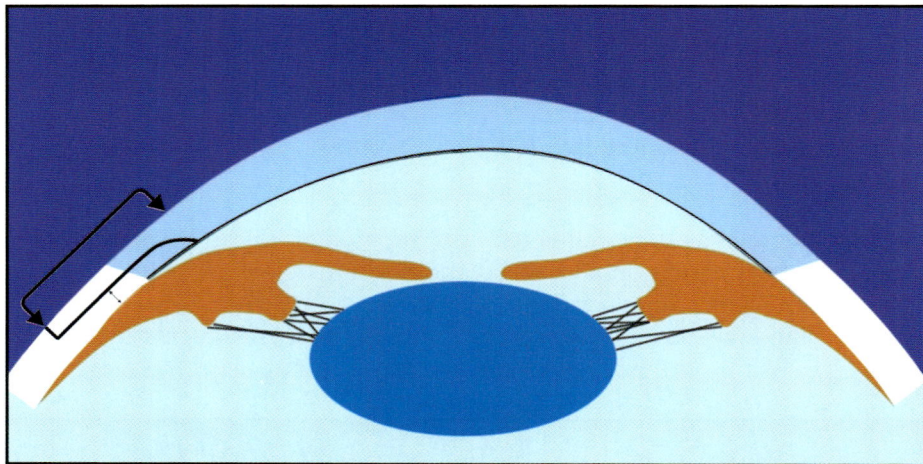

Fig. 7.8: Length of tunnel is shown by arrow

PROCEDURE FOR CONSTRUCTION OF TUNNEL

Sclerocorneal tunnel

Instruments needed:

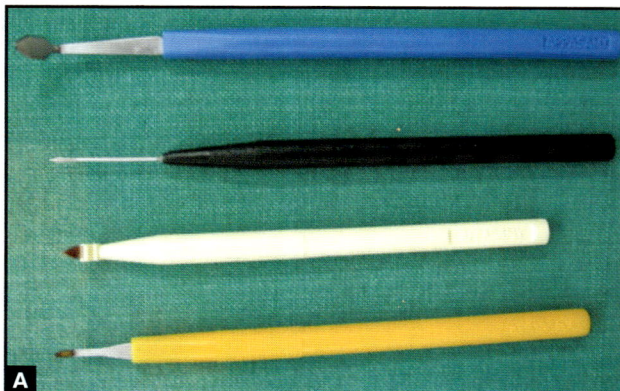

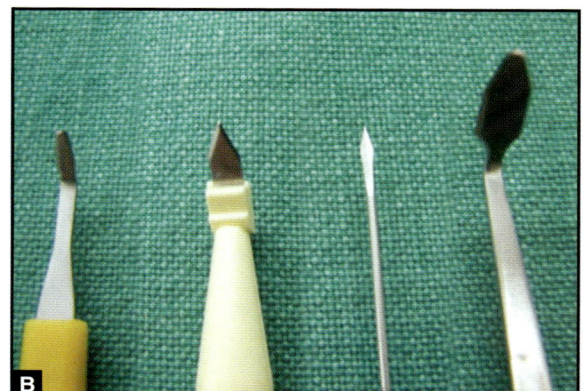

Figs 7.9A and B: Instruments for making tunnel incisions

Crescent knife, 2.8 keratome, sideport entry knife, 5.2 keratome.

- Diamond knife or metal knife with depth calibration
- Crescent knife with bevel up blade. Incision extension blade with bevel up.

Groove is made on the sclera up to a depth of 300 microns. Tunnel is made in the same depth in the sclera and the cornea upto a length of 2.5 mm (1.5 mm in sclera and 1mm in the cornea).

In clear corneal and near corneal incision

Instruments needed

- Diamond knife or metal knife with depth calibration
- Angled metal knife 2.8 mm.

It is always advisable to inject Viscoelastic through the paracentesis opening before making the tunnel incision. A groove is made to a depth of 300 microns and then a tunnel is made. The depth of the tunnel will be 2 mm.

Side Port Incision

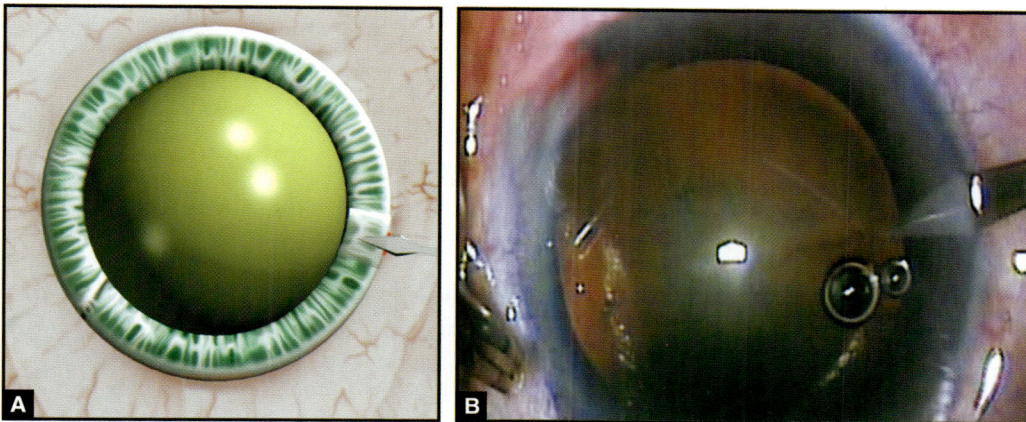

Fig. 7.10A and B: Side port incision

Uses

1. Injection of viscoelastic agents and irrigating fluid to maintain anterior chamber.
2. To perform maneuvers like nuclear rotation or nuclear fractures
3. Can be used to do capsulotomy by introducing needle through it
   Site of incision: Immediately anterior to the limbal vascular arcade at 10 O' clock or 2 O' clock.
   Size-About 1 mm.

One or two openings can be made depending on the type of cannula used for cortical clean up. If Simcoe is used, one port is sufficient but if bimanual irrigation and aspiration is used 2 openings will be required. Bimanual irrigation and aspiration is always ideal for cortical clean up.

8

Viscoelastics (Ocular viscosurgical devices - OVD)

With the advent of viscoelastic substances the quality of ophthalmic microsurgery has improved to a great extent. The complications occurring due to corneal endothelial damage have come down dramatically.

A viscoelastic substance has both viscous and elastic properties.

Viscosity is the ability of the substance to resist the stress forces while elasticity is the ability of the substance to alter its form when forces are applied and come back to its normal form when forces are removed.

Characteristics of ideal viscoelastic:

It should be inert and iso-osmotic
It should be non inflammatory and non toxic
It should be optically clear
Should not interfere with wound healing
It should have high viscosity to prevent damage to the intraocular tissues and to maintain spaces. Higher the molecular weight the more viscous the substance will be.

Uses of viscoelastics in cataract surgery:

1. To maintain anterior chamber and protect corneal endothelium during various steps as capsulotomy, nucleus expression, IOL insertion
2. To push the iris diaphragm back when there is vitreous upthrust
3. Management of detached descemet's membrane
4. To control intraocular bleeding during surgery.

Various viscoelastic substances available (Fig 8.1Ato C)

1. Hyaluronic acid
2. Methyl cellulose
3. Chondroitin sulphate
4. Polyacryl amide
5. Polytriethylene monomethacrylate
6. Collagen (Human placental collagen type IV).

Viscoelastics are of 2 types:

1. Cohesive
2. Adhesive (dispersive)

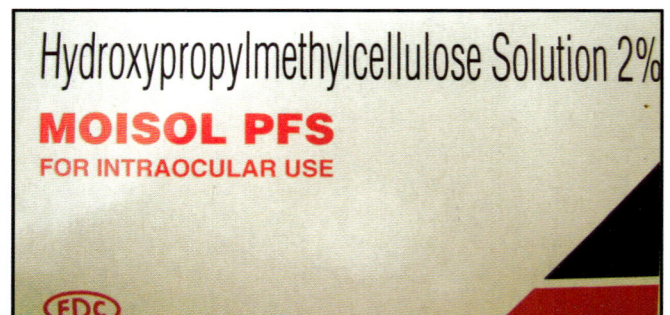

Fig. 8.1A: Hydroxypropyl methylcellulose

Viscoelastics (Ocular viscosurgical devices - OVD) **39**

1. Cohesive Viscoelastics: Derivatives of long chain hyaluronic acid

They have a high molecular weight.

Advantages

- Have great capacity to maintain spaces inside the eye and thus help in maintaining a deep anterior chamber
- Help in stabilizing the intraocular tissues like iris, capsule and vitreous
- Can be easily and rapidly aspirated at the end of surgery.

Disadvantages

- In phacosurgery due to complete removal from the anterior chamber, there is increased risk of corneal endothelial damage
- Residual substance may block the trabecular mesh work and cause secondary glaucoma
- Capsular distension syndrome is common if the substance is left behind the IOL.

Uses

- To maintain anterior chamber during the introduction of instruments
- To do a stable capsulorhexis
- To break adhesions (synechiae)
- To dilate the pupil
- To implant IOL.

Cohesive viscoelastics examples

a. Healon -5
b. Healon GV
c. Microvisc plus
d. Amvisc plus

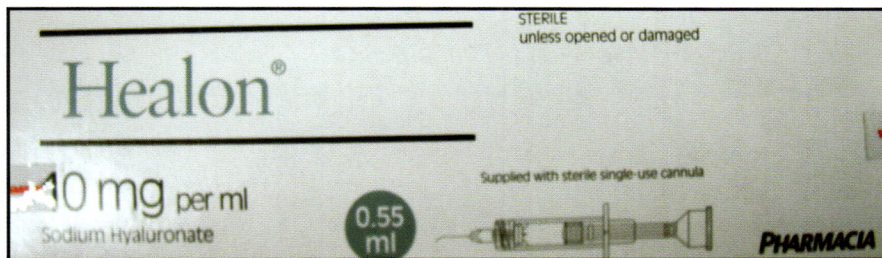

Fig. 8.1B: Sodium hyaluronidase

2. Dispersive Viscoelastics (Adhesive)

These are less cohesive and less viscous due to which they disperse rapidly in the anterior chamber.

Advantages:

- Less tendency to escape from anterior chamber and thus more protective to the endothelium
- Less risk of postoperative glaucoma
- Cost effective

Disadvantages

- Difficult to remove completely from anterior chamber
- Optically not as good as cohesive viscoelastics.

Dispersive Viscoelastics (Adhesive) examples

a. Methyl cellulose - Visco met, Moisol, Appa visc, Visilon
b. Chondroitin sulphate - Viscoat (Alcon)

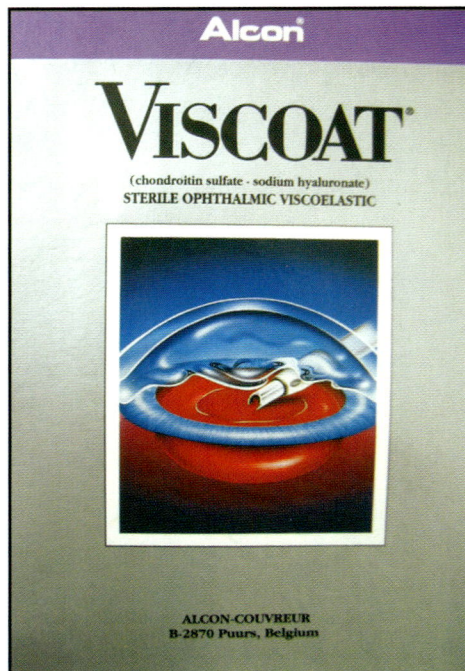

Fig. 8.1C: Chondroitin sulphate + sodium hyaluronate

It is to be remembered that the viscoelastic substances are not intraocular solutions but they are intraocular instruments which have to be removed completely at the end of surgery to avoid postoperative complications.

9

Intraocular Solutions

Ringer's lactate
Balanced salt solution (BSS)
Balanced salt solution plus (BSS Plus)

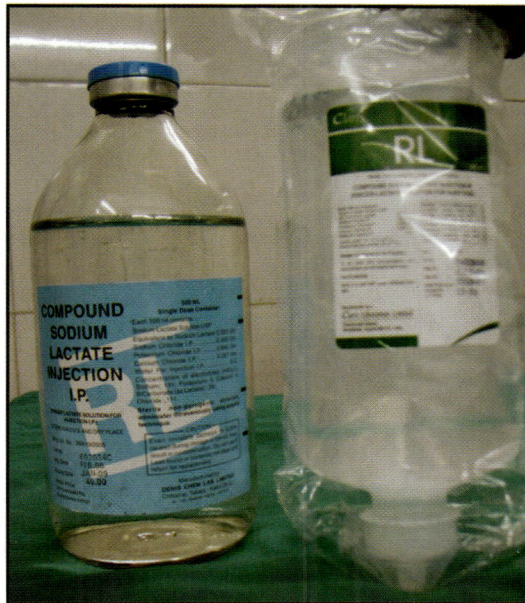

Fig. 9.1A: Ringer's lactate

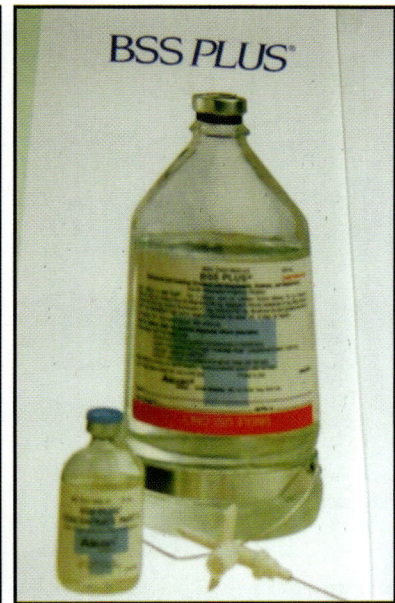

Fig. 9.1B: BSS plus

For routine cataract surgery with a short time procedure all three types of solutions can be used. For a long duration procedure and posterior segment surgeries it is preferable to use BSS or BSS plus.

Table 9.1: Composition of Ringer's lactate, BSS and BSS Plus solutions

Composition (mmol /L)	Ringer's Lactate	BSS	BSS plus
Sodium chloride	102	110	122.2
Potassium chloride	4	10	5.08
Calcium chloride	3	3	1.05
Sodium bicarbonate	-	-	25
Sodium acetate	-	29	-
Sodium lactate	28	-	-
Sodium citrate	-	6	-
Glucose	-	-	5.11
Glutathione	-	-	0.33
Osmolality	277	305	305
pH	6-7.2	7.4	7.4

10

Capsular Incision (Capsulotomy)

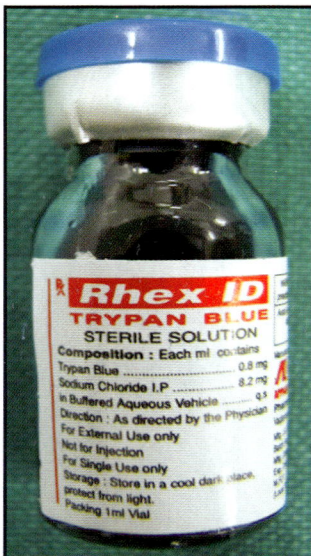

Fig. 10.1A: Trypan blue dye for staining the capsule

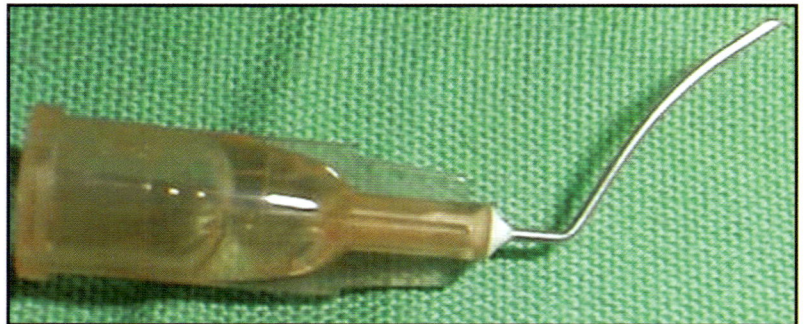

Fig. 10.1B: Cystitome needle (bent 26G needle)

Types of capsulotomies

1. Can opener capsulotomy
2. Envelope capsulotomy
3. Continuous curvilinear capsulorhexis
4. R.F capsulotomy

1. Can opener capsulotomy

It is done with a bent 26 gauge needle. Radial cuts are made in the anterior capsule all round 360 degrees and the capsule is opened. This type of capsulotomy is done in conventional ECCE and SICS.

I prefer postal stamp technique of can opener capsulotomy in which 60-70 punctures are made in the capsule and joined by which a predetermined capsulotomy size with minimal tags and simulates that of capsulorhexis.

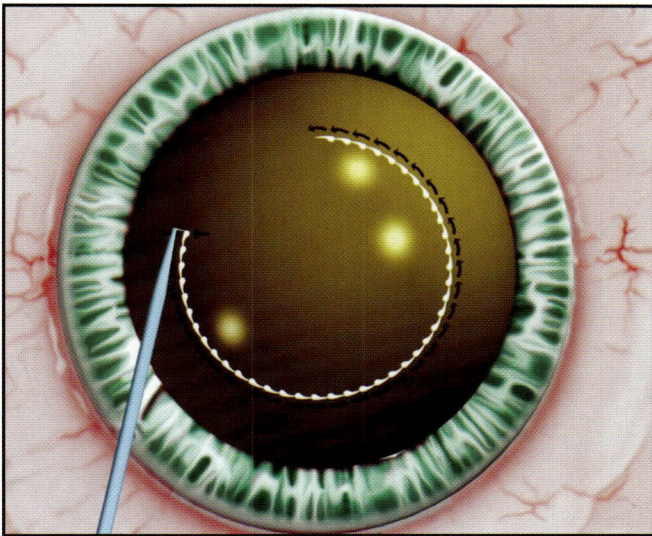

Fig. 10.2A: Can opener capsulotomy

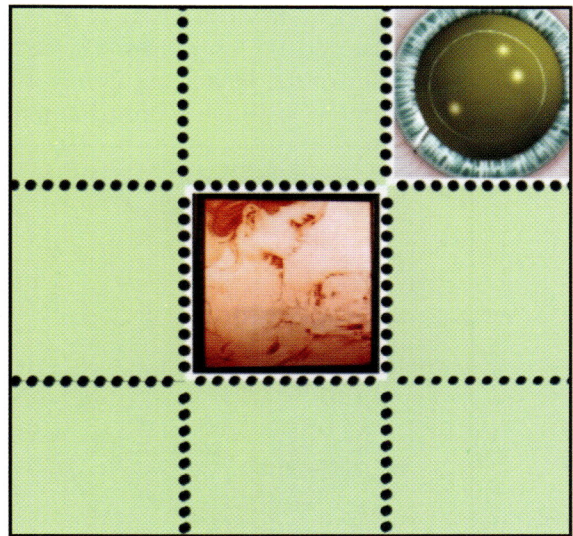

Fig. 10.2B: Postal stamp technique of can opener capsulotomy -multiple holes weaken the capsule and open it up

Disadvantages of can opener capsulotomy

- In the bag IOL implantation is not possible leading to decentration
- Posterior capsular opacification is more common
- Posterior extension of capsulotomy results in posterior capsular rent.

Advantages

- Easy to learn
- Preferable in very hard and large nucleus in non phaco cases.

2. **Envelope capsulotomy:** A linear opening is made in the anterior capsule from 2 O' clock to 10 O' clock position. Then the nucleus is expressed through the capsular incision. Endocapsular cortical clean up is done. IOL is implanted in the bag. The anterior capsule is cut to the predetermined size.

Advantages

Endothelial damage during cortical clean up and IOL insertion can be minimized.

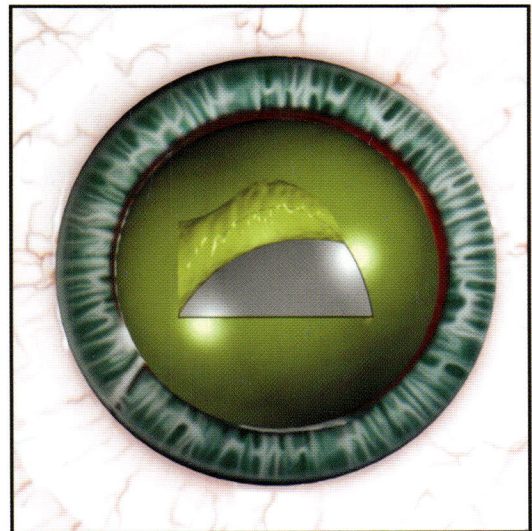

Fig. 10.2C: Envelope technique useful in hypermature cataracts

3. **Continuous curvilinear capsulorhexis (CCC):** It is the best type of capsulotomy. It can be done with a cystitome needle or capsulorhexis forceps.

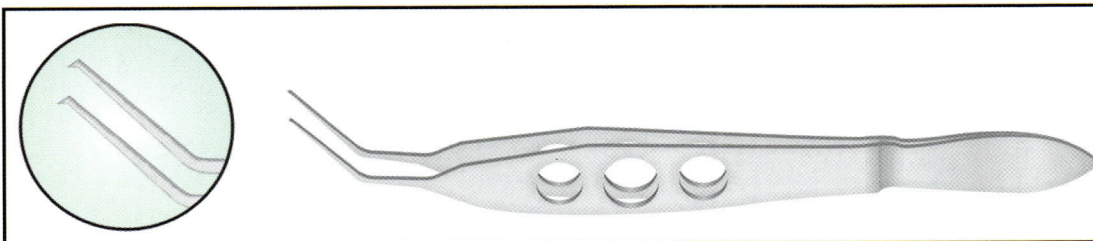

Fig. 10.3A: Capsulorhexis foceps

Before learning how to do CCC it is important to know the anatomy of the lens capsule. Posterior zonular fibers are inserted 1-1.5 mm from the equator. The anterior zonular fibers are inserted 2 mm from the equator. The diameter of the lens is about 9.5 -10 mm. So the area on the anterior lens capsule which is free from zonular attachment is above 6 mm diameter. So CCC has to be done in this area only.

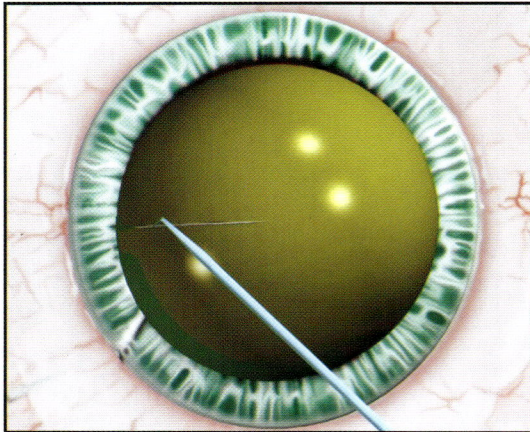

Fig. 10.3B: First step in making CCC

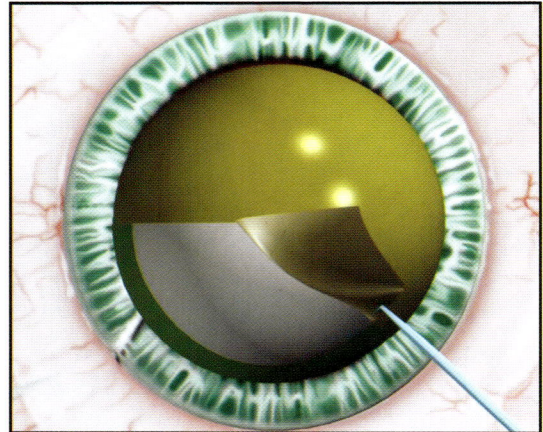

Fig. 10.3C: Diagram of CCC in the way

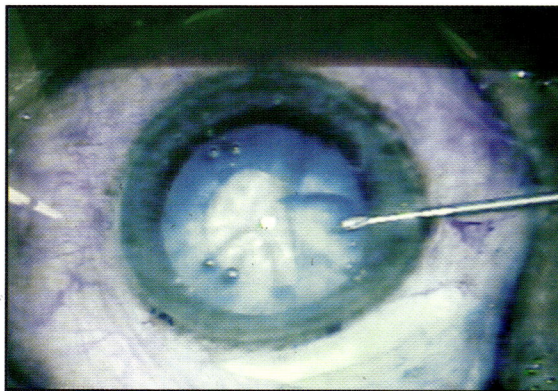

Fig. 10.3D: 3 CCC in the way

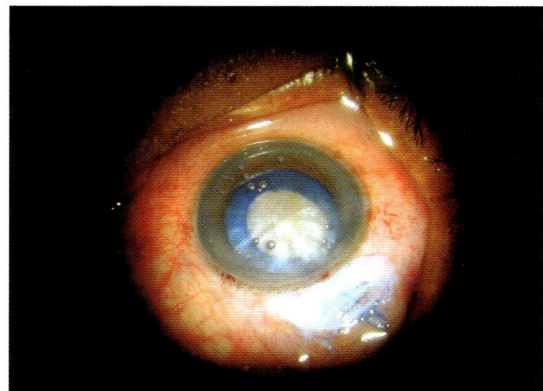

Fig. 10.3E: 4 after completion of CCC

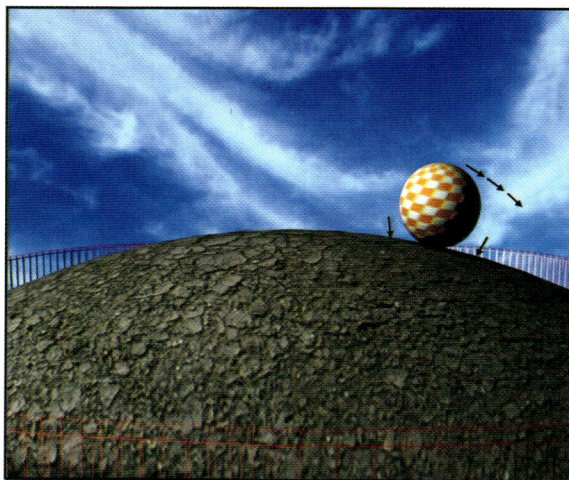

Fig. 10.3F: If the posterior capsule surface is convex as shown, there is a chance circular of CCC to run

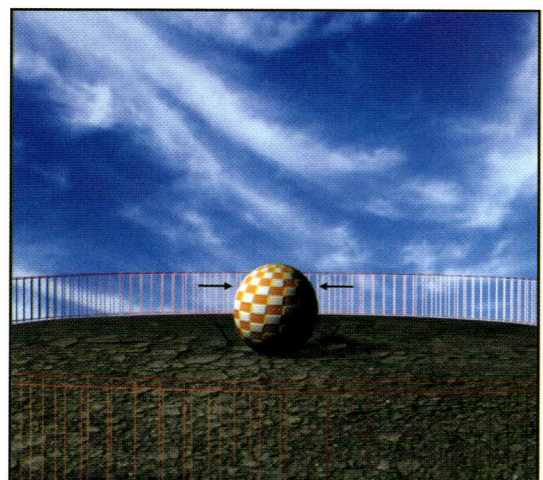

Fig. 10.3G: If posterior capsule is flat a stable rhexis can be made as we see deep AC

Performed by 2 techniques

1. Shearing

2. Ripping

1. *Shearing techniques:* The force is applied in the same direction of the tear and is minimal.

2. *Ripping:* The force is applied not only in the same plane but also perpendicular to the direction of the tear. The force applied will be more.

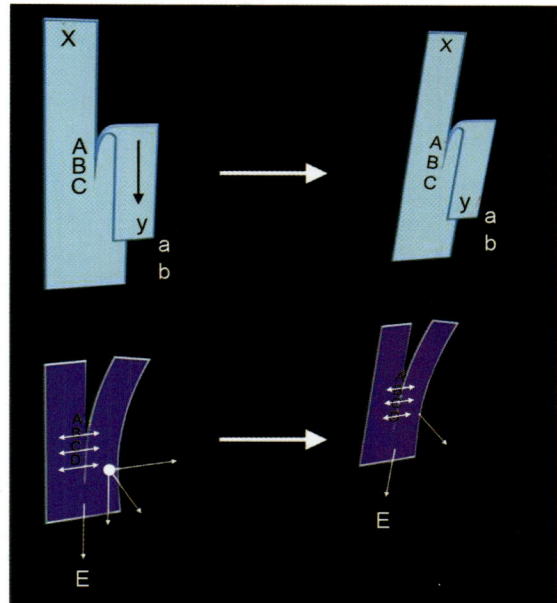

Fig. 10.3H: CCC techniques shearing and ripping

Advantages of CCC

- In the bag phacoemulsification can be done
- Implantation of IOL in the bag is well facilitated, decreasing the incidence of decentration and PCO formation
- CCC facilitates easy cortical clean up due to absence of tags
- In cases of posterior capsule rupture, rim of the CCC acts as a support for the IOL placed in the sulcus
- In the postoperative period the risk of IOL contact with the ciliary body and iris will be absent, thereby less postoperative inflammation, hyphema and pigment dispersion is caused.

Complications of CCC

- Capsular contraction syndrome
- Capsular bag hyperdistension
- Epithelial cell proliferation on the posterior capsule

  Dimensions of CCC: It should be about 5-6 mm. Small or big rhexis leads to problems.

Small rhexis–Problems

- Phacoemulsification and implantation of IOL will be difficult
- Postoperatively examination of peripheral retina becomes difficult due to opacification of anterior capsule rim
- Increased risk of phimosis of capsular bag.

Big rhexis - Problems

- The nuclear fragments come out of the capsular bag during phaco.

Posterior capsulorhexis

It is done in cases of small posterior capsule ruptures to avoid extension towards the periphery. This is done commonly in children to avoid posterior capsular opacification which may be difficult to manage later.

(has to be done in pediatric cataract to prevent PCO)

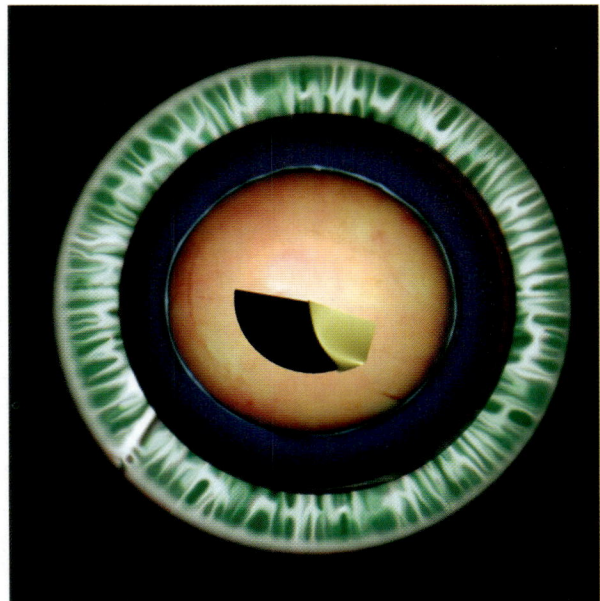

Fig. 10.3I: Posterior capsulorhexis

Capsulorhexis in difficult situations

In mature cataract:

- Due to absence of red glow visualization of capsule will be difficult. In these cases capsule can be stained using Trypan blue which enhances the visibility. It can alter the behavior of the capsule.

Hypermature cataract:

After puncturing the capsule all the cortical matter should be flushed out with viscoelastic substance and capsular bag filled with viscoelastic and then capsulorhexis is done.

RF capsulotomy:

It is done using radio frequency probe useful in pediatric cataracts where the capsule is highly elastic.

11

Hydroprocedures

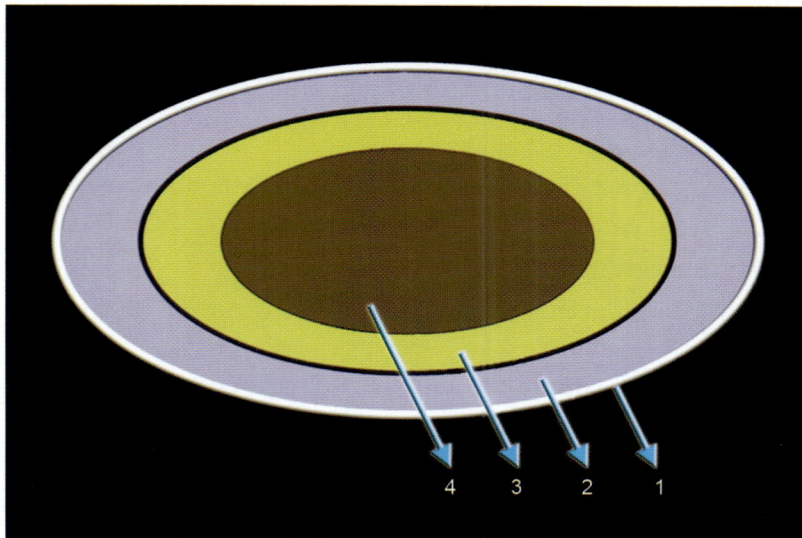

Fig. 11.1: Different layers of the lens (1.capsule 2.cortex 3. epinucleus 4. nucleus)

Hydrodissection: Injection of irrigating fluid (BSS or Ringer's lactate) below the anterior capsule with a blunt and flat tipped cannula. (Hydrodissection cannula) attached to a 1 CC syringe which separates the cortex from the epinucleus of the lens.

- First decompression of anterior chamber is done by removing excess viscoelastic before doing hydrodissection.
- 26 or 27 gauge blunt flat tipped cannula is used to do hydrodissection to avoid damage to the capsule.
- Injection of fluid done at one place will be sufficient most of the times. If it is not sufficient, injection and simultaneous mechanical rotation for decompression has to be done.
- Fluid should be injected steadily using sufficient force. Too much force should not be used as it may damage the posterior capsule.
- After complete hydrodissection the nucleus freely rotates under the anterior capsule.

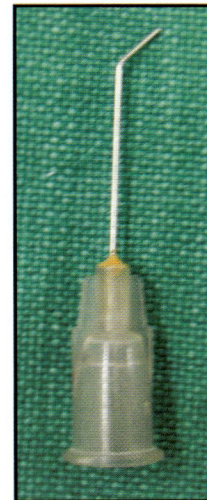

Fig. 11.2: Hydrodissection cannula

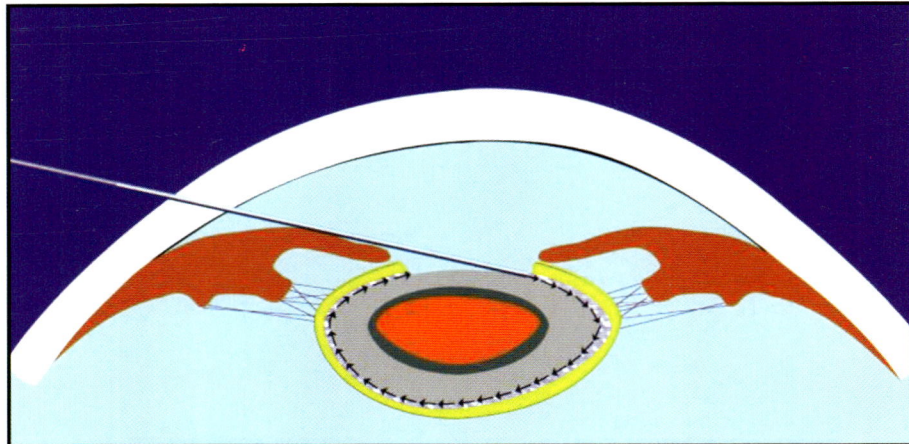

Fig. 11.3: Hydrodissection fluid passes under the capsule

Hydrodissection is a very important step in cases of immature cataract where the cortex which is closely adherent to the epinucleus gets separated. In mature and hypermature cataracts most of the cortex will be loose, so minimal or no hydrodissection is required.

In cases of posterior polar cataracts hydrodissection should not be done as it will damage the posterior capsule.

Hydrodelineation or Hydrodelamination

This is a procedure in which the epinucleus is separated from the central dense nucleus by the injection of fluid into the superficial layers of the lens.

- The tip of the cannula is introduced into the superficial layers of the lens and fluid is injected.
- The tip of the cannula should be passed sufficiently under the anterior capsule so that the fluid is directed towards the equator of the lens.
- The separation of nucleus from the epinucleus will be seen as a golden ring appearance.
- In soft cataract hydrodelineation may be continued even till 1 to 2 or 3 golden rings are seen.

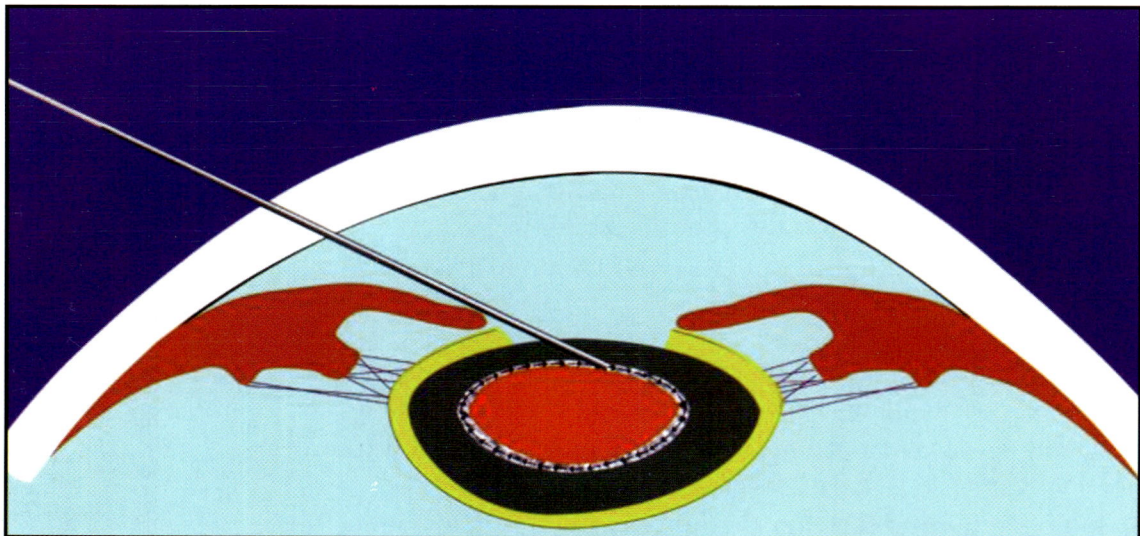

Fig. 11.4A: Hydrodelineation (fluid passes between epinucleus and nucleus)

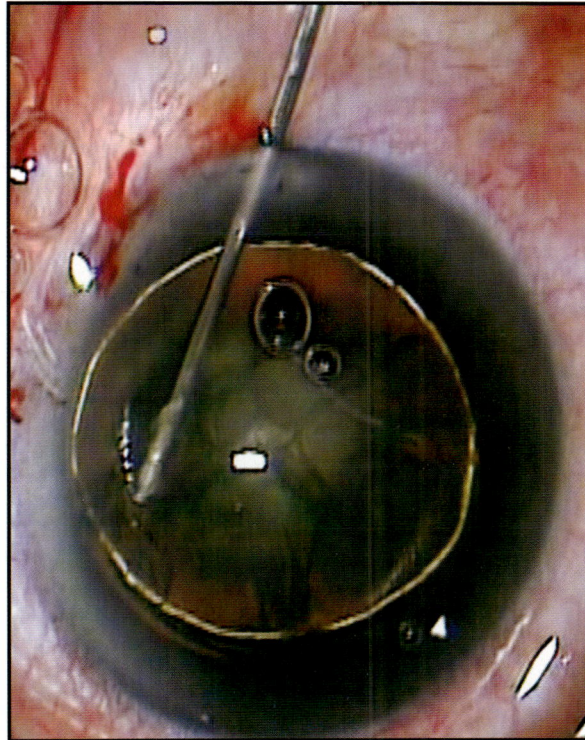

Fig. 11.4B: Golden ring appearance

Hydrodelineation is an important step in phacoemulsification surgery.

In small incision cataract surgery by hydrodelineation the size of the nucleus can be reduced due to separation of epinucleus.

Advantages of hydroprocedures:

- Easy mobilization of nucleus.
- Protection of the capsule and zonule while managing the nucleus.
- The size of the nucleus is reduced by separating it from superficial epinuclear layers.

Section

2

12

Nucleus Management in SICS

Nucleus prolapsed into the anterior chamber.

Nucleus delivery or removal.

- Nucleus prolapse should be done into the anterior chamber after separation of the nucleus by good hydrodissection and hydrodelineation. It can be done by various methods:

1. Hydroprocedure it self may prolapse the nucleus into the AC.

2. Nucleus may be dialed with the same hydrodissection cannula so that a part of the equator is prolapsed out of the capsular bag. The remaining part may be dialed out after injecting viscoelastic with the tip of the same cannula (The author prefers this procedure).

3. After injecting viscoelastic into the anterior chamber the nucleus pressed at one side at 9 O' clock which lifts the nucleus on other side at 3 O' clock position. The nucleus is then rotated with the tip of the cannula into the anterior chamber.

4. Rotating the nucleus with using a Sinskey's hook. The iris is retracted at 12 O' clock position and with the hook the nucleus tipped and rotated.

5. In mature and hypermature cataracts after completing capsulotomy the same needle may be used to rotate the nucleus out of the capsular bag.

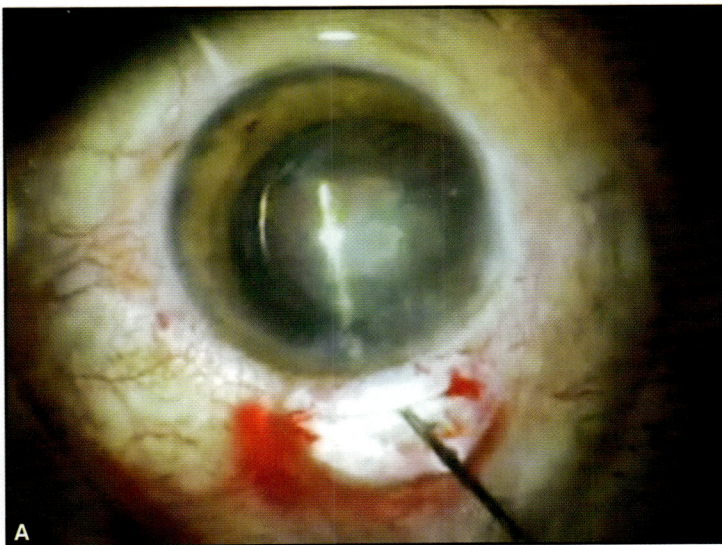

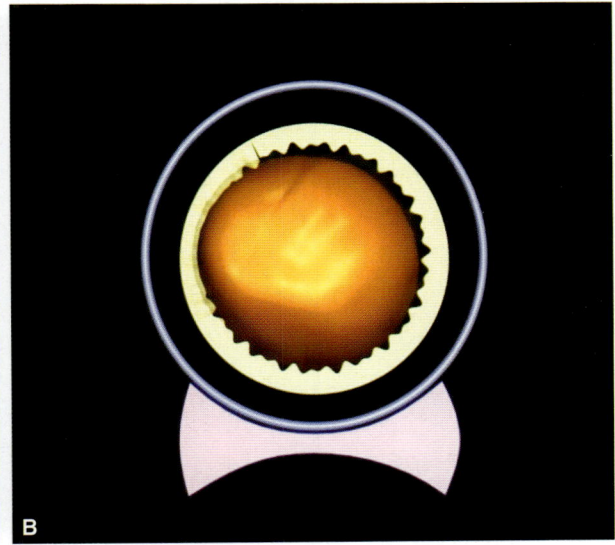

Figs 12.1A and B: Nucleus prolapsed into anterior chamber

Problems in prolapsing the nucleus into the AC

- *Small pupil:* Manual dilatation of pupil or multiple sphincterotomies are done
- *Small CCC:* Radial relaxing cuts have to be made in the anterior capsule
- *Incomplete capsulotomy:* Complete capsulotomy can be done by using trypan blue dye for enhancing the visibility of the capsule
- *Posterior syncline:* They have to be separated by passing a fine iris spatula under the iris all around.

13

Nucleus Removal or Delivery

Various methods

1. Viscoexpression technique
2. Wire vectis techniques
3. Irrigating vectis
4. Nucleus sandwich technique
5. Bluementhal technique
6. Nucleus fracture technique
7. Fish hook technique.

Viscoexpression technique

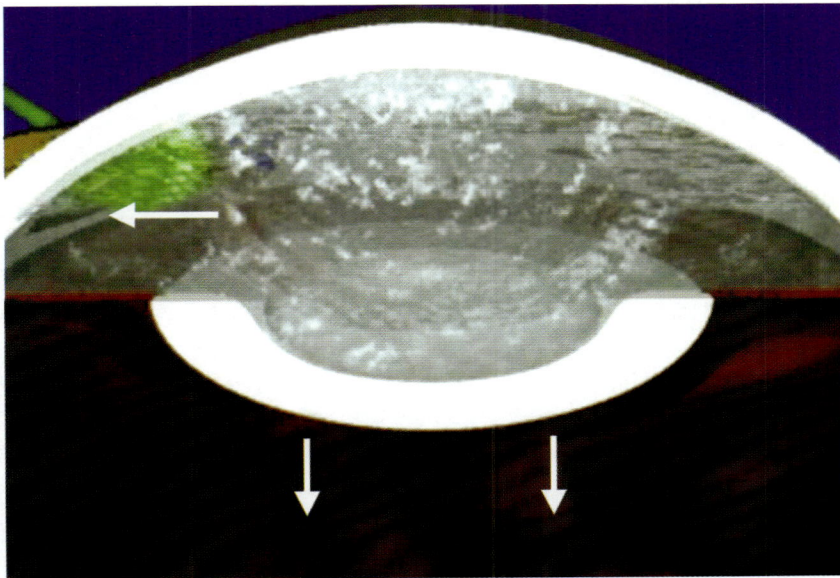

Fig. 13.1A: Viscoexpression (*Note:* The viscopushes the posterior capsule deep and also protects the endothelium).

Viscocannula should be passed under the nucleus upto 6 O' clock position and gradually pressurize the chamber by injecting viscoelastic. At the same time posterior scleral lip is depressed. The nucleus slowly slides out of the tunnel. Before doing this, good hydrodelineation should be done and the nucleus must be well separated from the outer epinucleus.

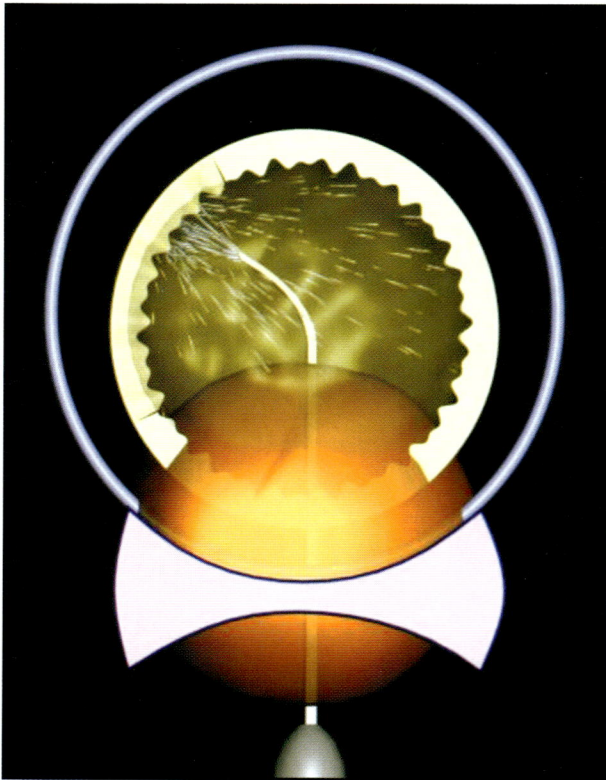

Fig. 13.1B: Viscoexpression

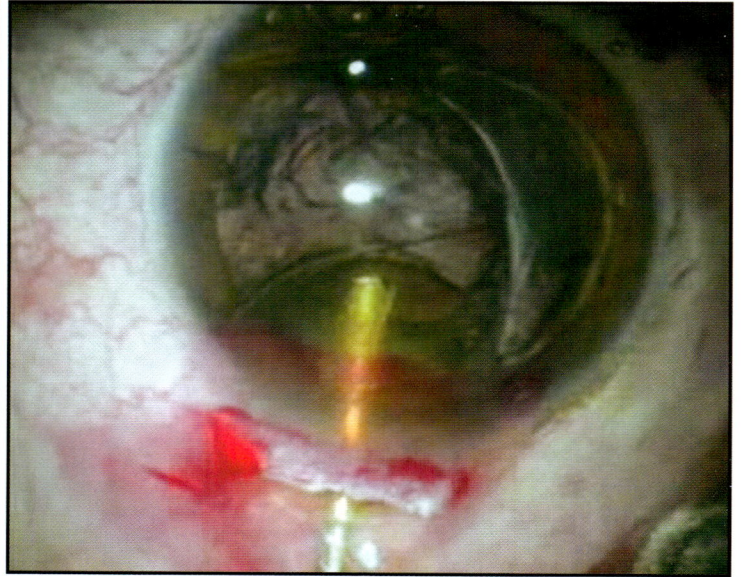

Fig. 13.1C: Nucleus being expressed

Wire Vectis Technique

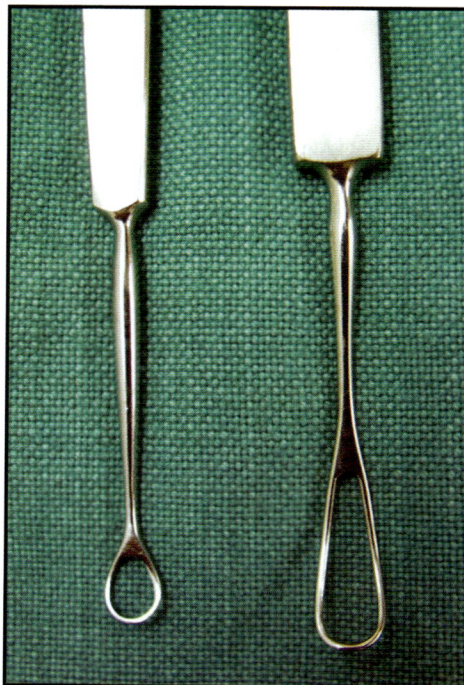

Fig. 13.2A: A wire vectis and long vectis

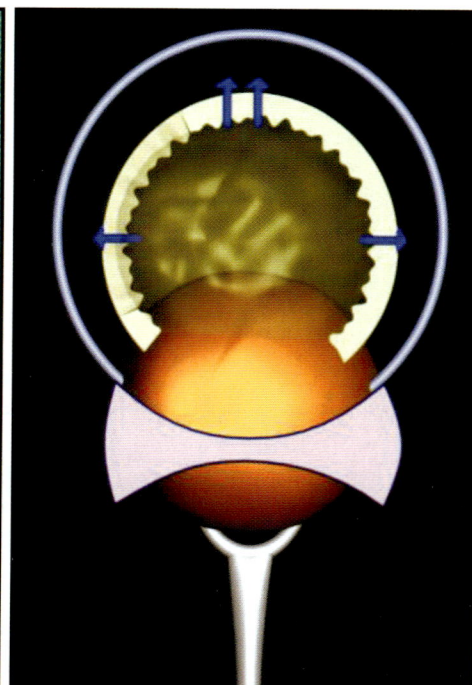

Fig. 13.2B: Vectis removal of nucleus

Long vectis is better than short one

After prolapsing the nucleus into the AC some viscoelastic is injected above and below the nucleus and wire vectis is passed under the nucleus. Slight traction is applied, at the same time depressing the posterior scleral lip with the shaft of the vectis. The nucleus comes out and epinucleus is removed by viscoexpression. This procedure is easy to perform.

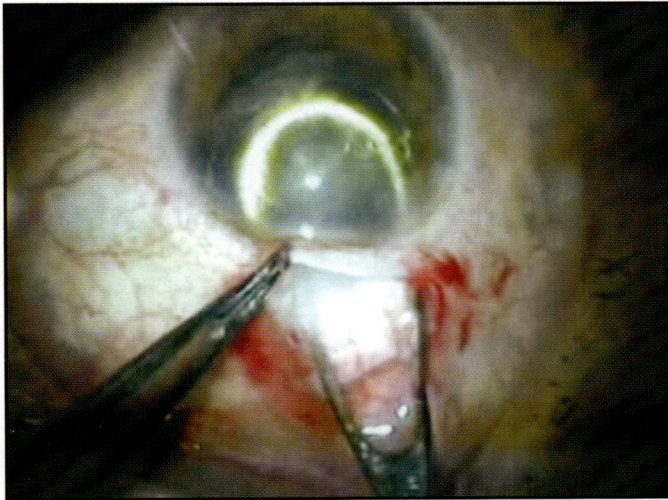

Fig. 13.2C: Vectis removal
(make sure that the vectis is not engaging the inferior iris)

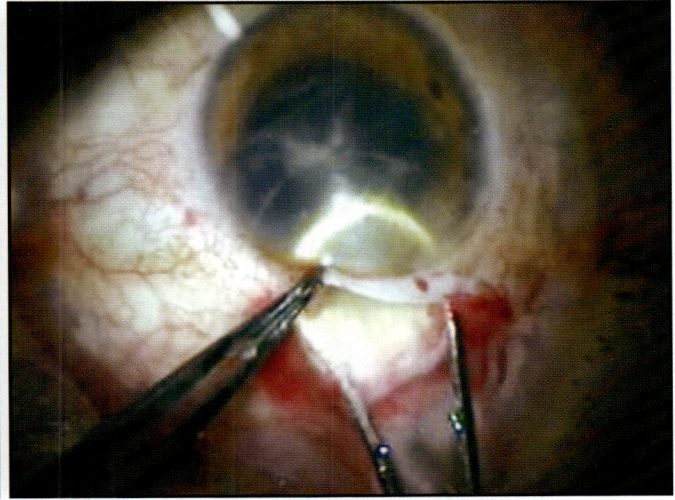

Fig. 13.2D: Vectis removal
(size of the incision should be such that it accommodates the nucleus)

Corneal endothelial damage can be prevented by liberal use of viscoelastic.

Care should be taken not to include the inferior iris between the nucleus and vectis as it may cause inferior iridodialysis. This can be prevented by injecting viscoelastic underneath the nucleus.

Irrigating Vectis

After prolapsing the nucleus into the anterior chamber, the irrigating vectis with the flow on is introduced under the nucleus and slowly expressed out of the tunnel by applying traction and depressing the posterior scleral lip.

Nucleus sandwich technique

After prolapsing the nucleus into the anterior chamber, viscoelastic is injected above and below the nucleus. The wire vectis is passed under the nucleus and Sinskeys hook is passed over the nucleus and the nucleus is gripped between the two instruments and is delivered by applying traction.

Bluementhal technique

In this technique, while making the tunnel incision, scleral pockets are created to accommodate the nucleus while it slides out of the wound. An anterior chamber maintainer is inserted in to the AC from the inferior limbus. Continuous irrigation helps in maintaining a deep anterior chamber and at the same time the pressure of the fluid pushes the nucleus out of the tunnel at the superior limbus. A silicone glide (spatula) introduced for easy delivery of the nucleus as it guides the nucleus out and also prevents iris prolapse through the wound.

Nucleus fracture technique

After prolapsing the nucleus into the anterior chamber a viscoelastic is injected above and below the nucleus. A vectis is introduced underneath the nucleus using a bisector or a trisector steady pressure is applied over

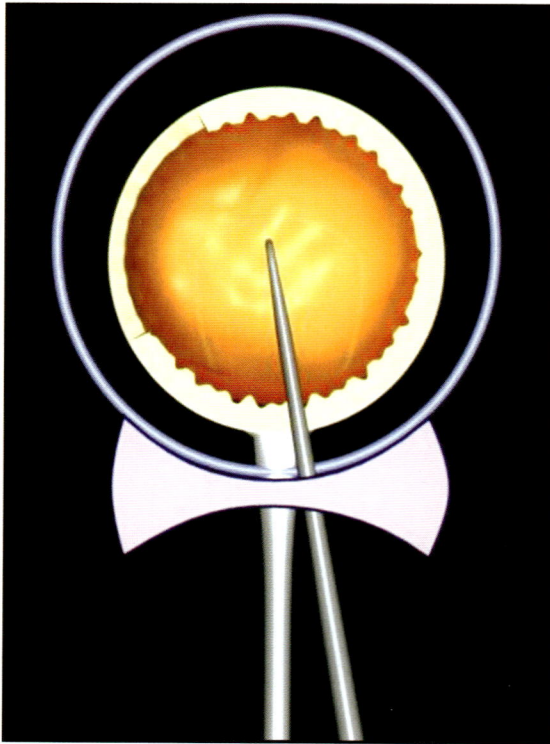

Fig. 13.3A: Sandwich technique: Vectis is kept under the nucleus and Sinskey's hook over the nucleus

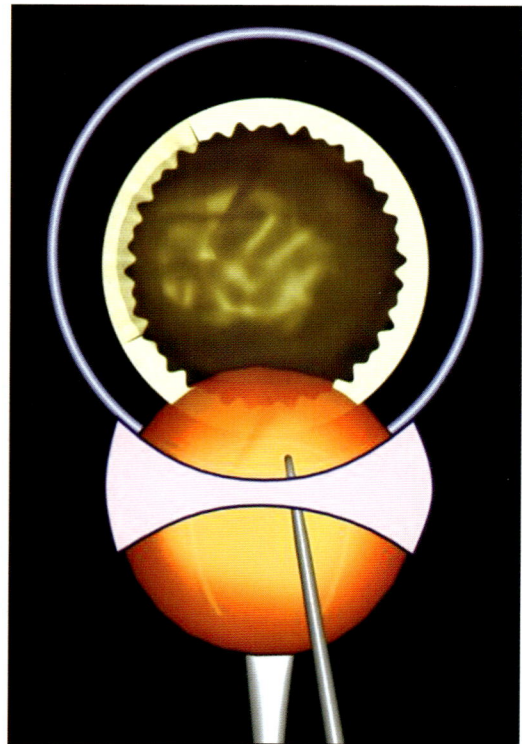

Fig. 13.3B: Sandwich technique: The nucleus is gripped between the two instruments and delivered out

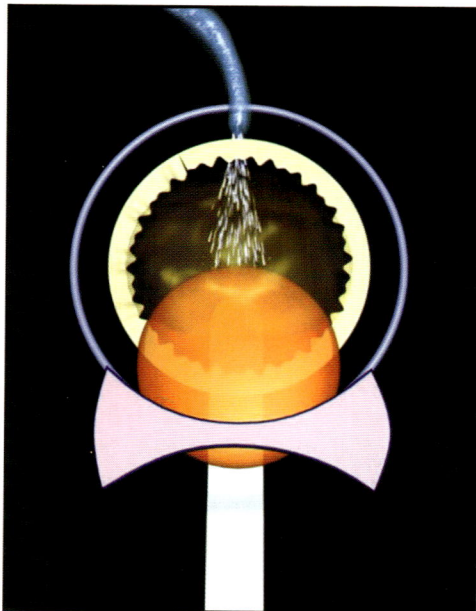

Fig. 13.4: Bluementhal technique: AC maintainer is put in at 6 O' clock position

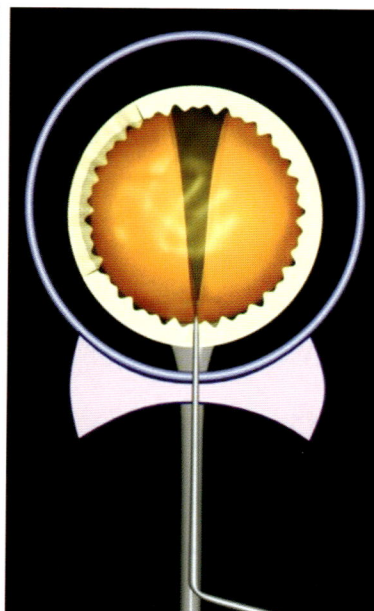

Fig. 13.5A: Nucleus fragmented into two halves using bisector

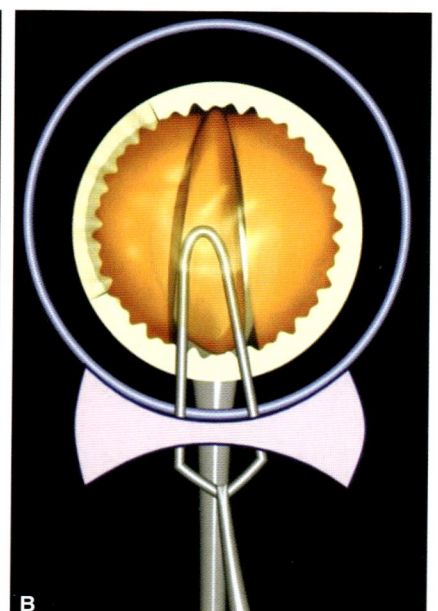

Fig. 13.5B: Nucleus is fragmented into 3 pieces using trisector

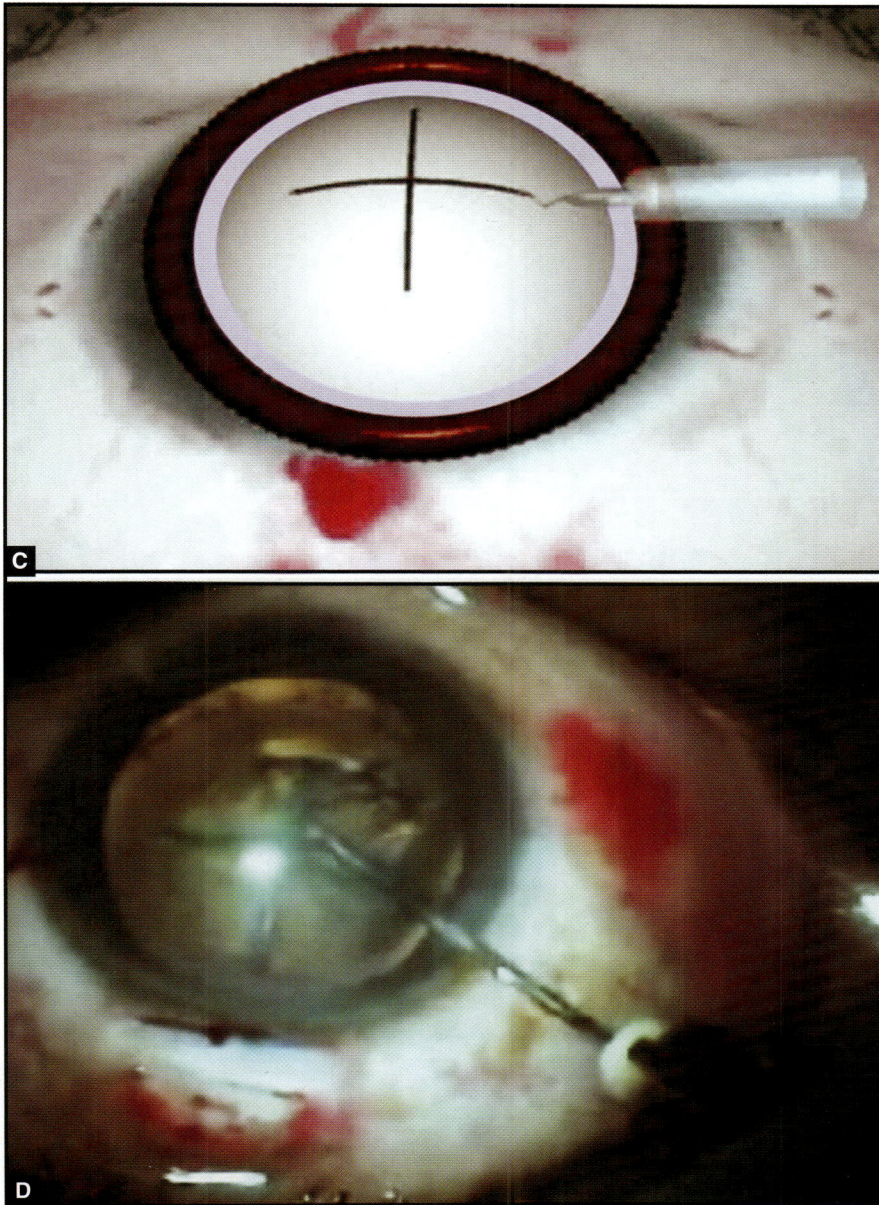

Figs 13.5C and D: Cruciate groove made with a cystitome

the nucleus so that it is broken into two or three fragments and these fragments are removed by visco expression.

A method of nucleus fracture (Authors modification) after anterior capsulotomy. A cruciate groove is created with a cystitome in the hard nucleus after which hydroprocedure is carried out then the viscoelastic is injected in to the AC and nucleus is fragmented using 2 choppers bimanually.

Then the fragments are removed by viscoexpression.

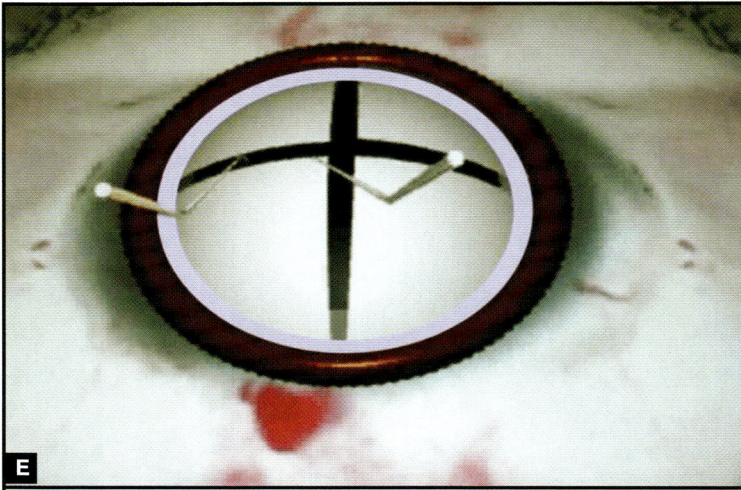

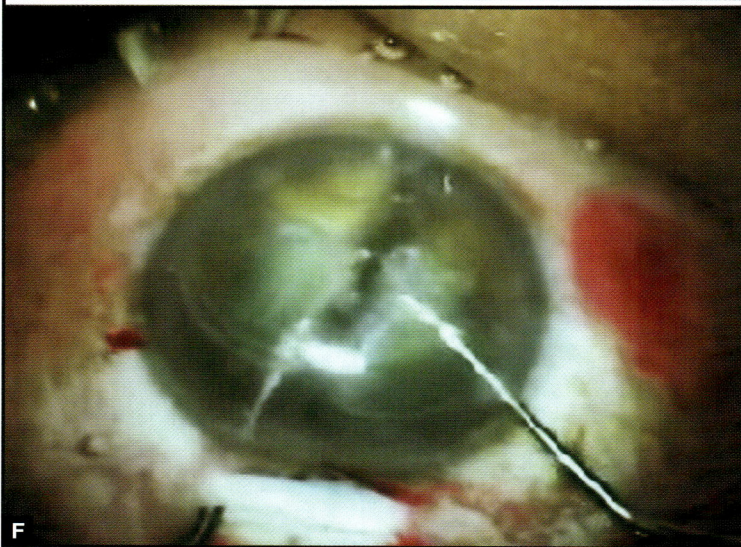

Figs 13.5E and F: Nucleus fragmented into four quadrants using two choppers

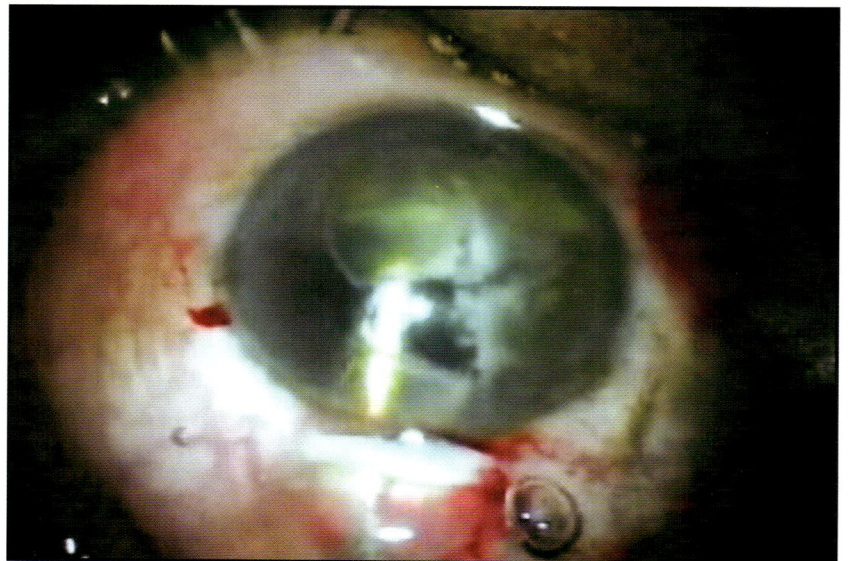

Fig. 13.5G: Fragments delivered by visco expression

Fracture in the tunnel: A large nucleus is engaged in the tunnel. The outer one-third of the nucleus is fractured within the tunnel with the help of microvectis with a square edge. The nucleus is levered within the tunnel. The outer one-third of the nucleus will come out. The remainings is pushed back into the AC with the help of viscoelastic and rotated to its longitudinal axis and delivered by the same vectis or by visco expression.

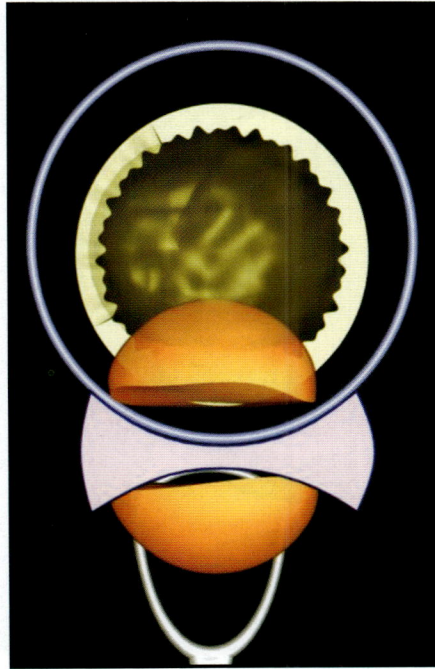

Fig. 13.6A: Fracture of nucleus in the tunnel

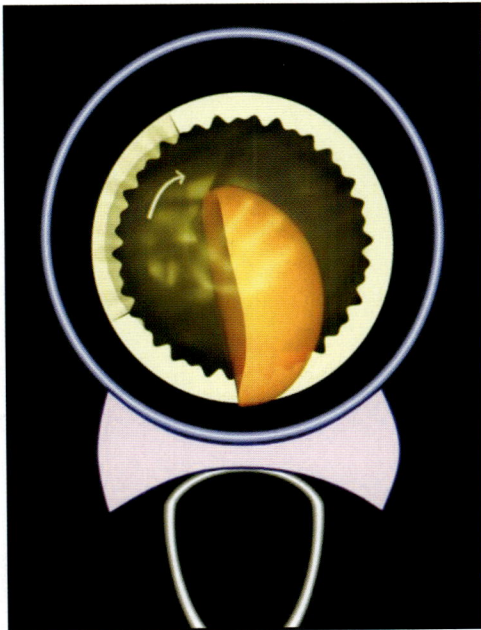

Fig. 13.6B: Residual fragment pushed into AC and aligned vertically

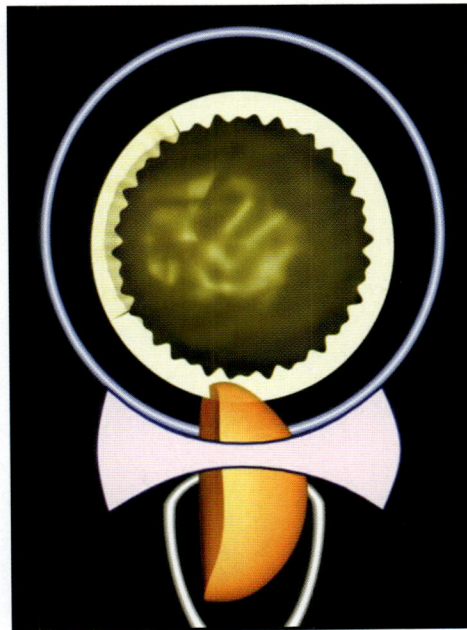

Fig. 13.6C: Residual fragment is removed

Fish hook technique: In this technique an envelope type of capsulotomy is made and the upper pole of the nucleus is rotated out after hydroprocedures. Viscoelastic is injected above and below the nucleus and a 30 sG disposable needle with the tip bent in the form of a fish hook is introduced under the nucleus and the lower pole of the nucleus is hooked and delivered out gently.

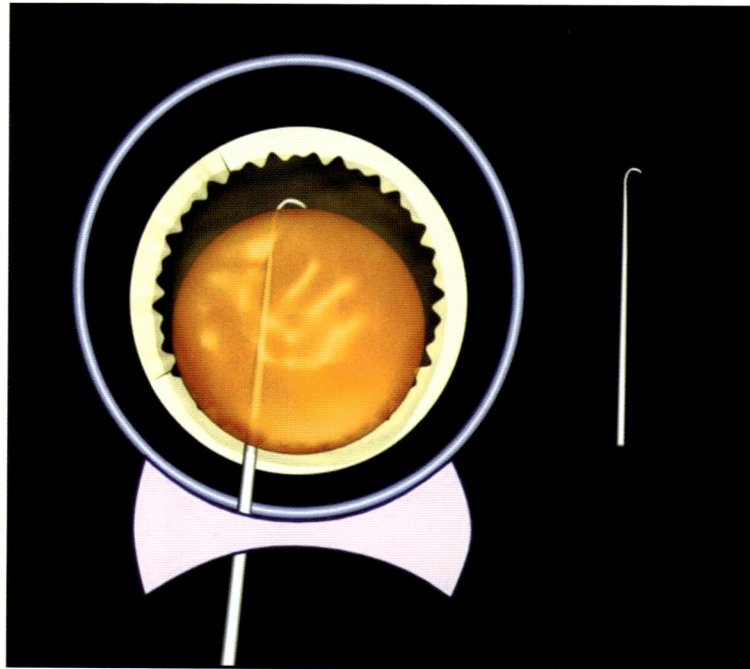

Fig. 13.7: Fish hook technique (Bent cystitome is passed under the nucleus and it is hooked and removed)

14

Cortical Clean Up

1. **Manual with Simcoe cannula**
   Regular
   Reverse
   J cannula for 12 O' clock cortical clean up

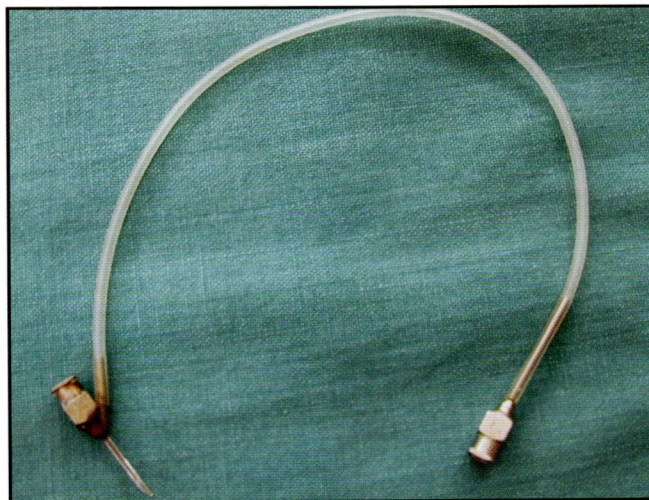

Fig. 14.1A: Simcoe cannula for manual I and A in SICS

2. **Automated system**
   Coaxial
   Bimanual

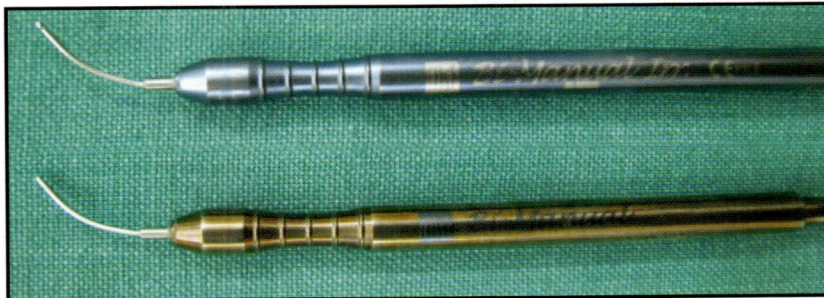

Fig. 14.1B: Bimanual I and A

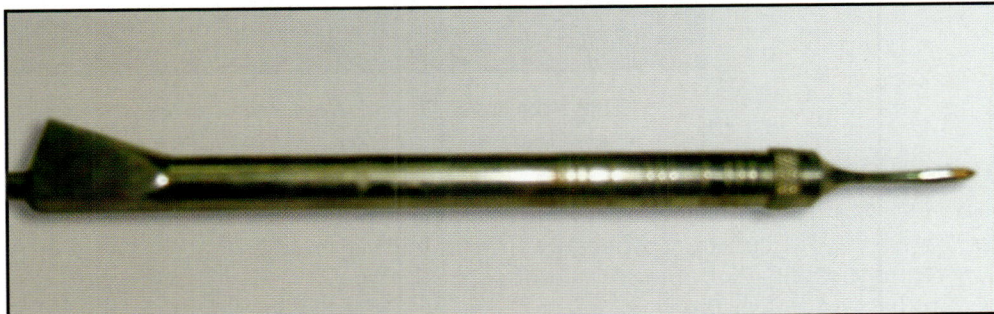

Fig. 14.1C: Co-axial I and A used in phacosurgery

Manual

Authors prefer reverse Simcoe where the eyebrow will not come in the way of the aspiration syringe. It also affords good maneuverability and enables good control of aspiration with the left hand.

12 O' clock cortex can be aspirated from the side port rather than the "J" cannula.

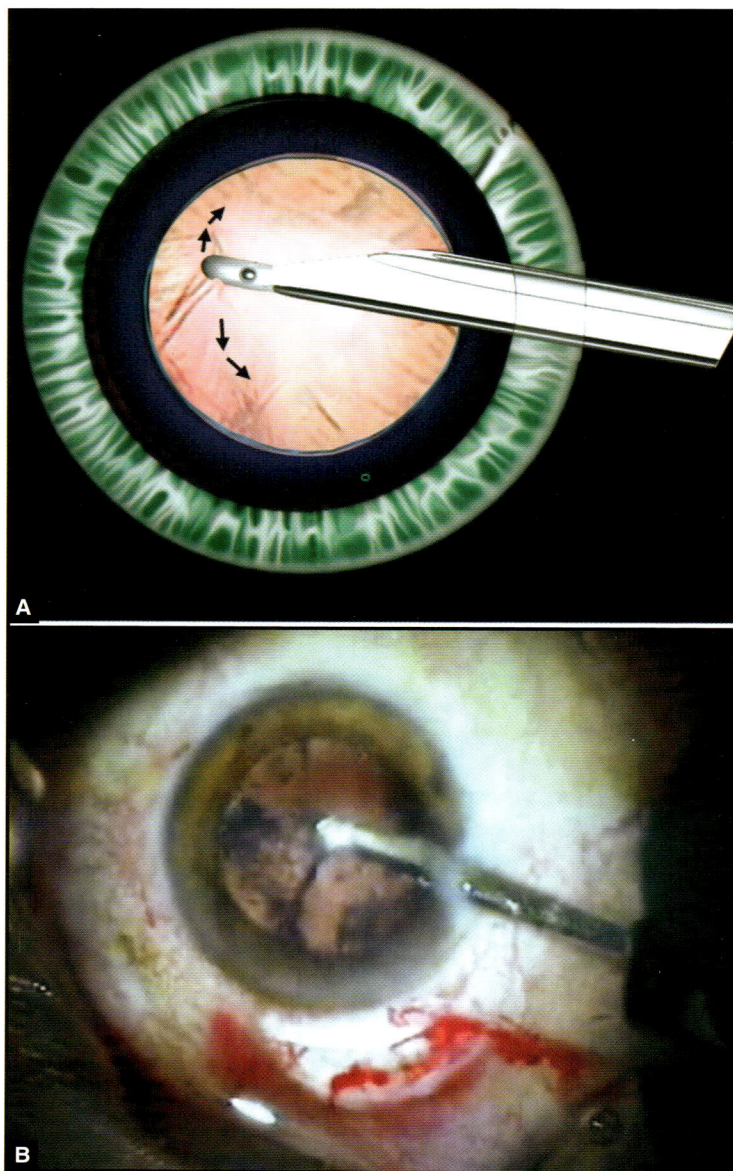

Figs 14.2A and B: Cortical aspiration using simcoe cannula

Automated

Coaxial system: With phacoemulsification irrigation and aspiration probe.
Disadvantages: Difficult to aspirate 12 O' clock cortical matter.

Frequent collapse of anterior chamber

Not easy to polish the capsule

Bimanual

Advantages: Easy to approach all the 360°.

Well-maintained anterior chamber and capsular bag.

Capsular polishing is easy.

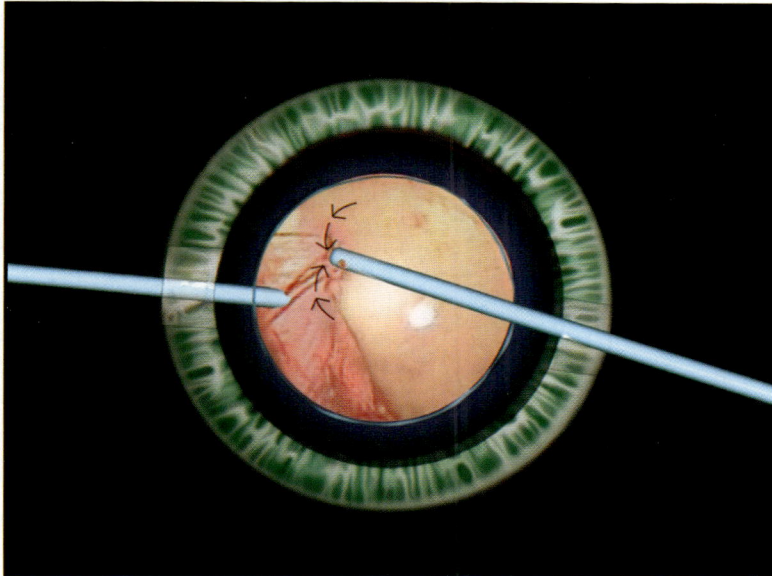

Fig. 14.2C: Cortical clean up with bimanual I and A

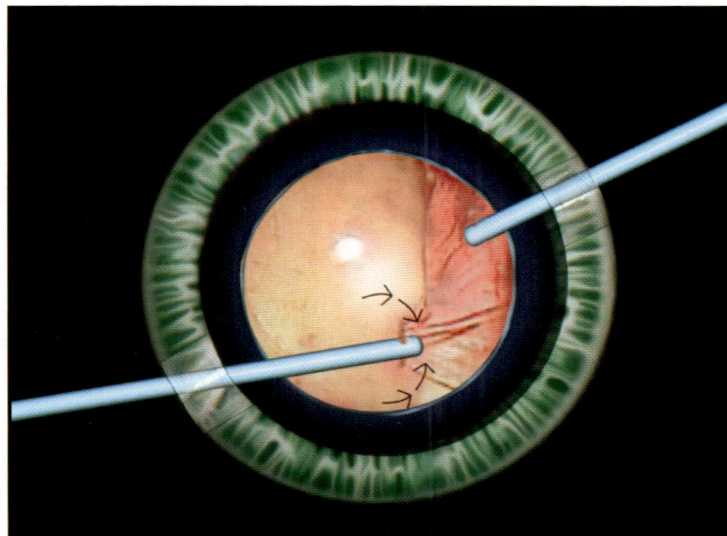

Fig. 14.2D: Cortical clean up of remaining half by interchanging the cannula

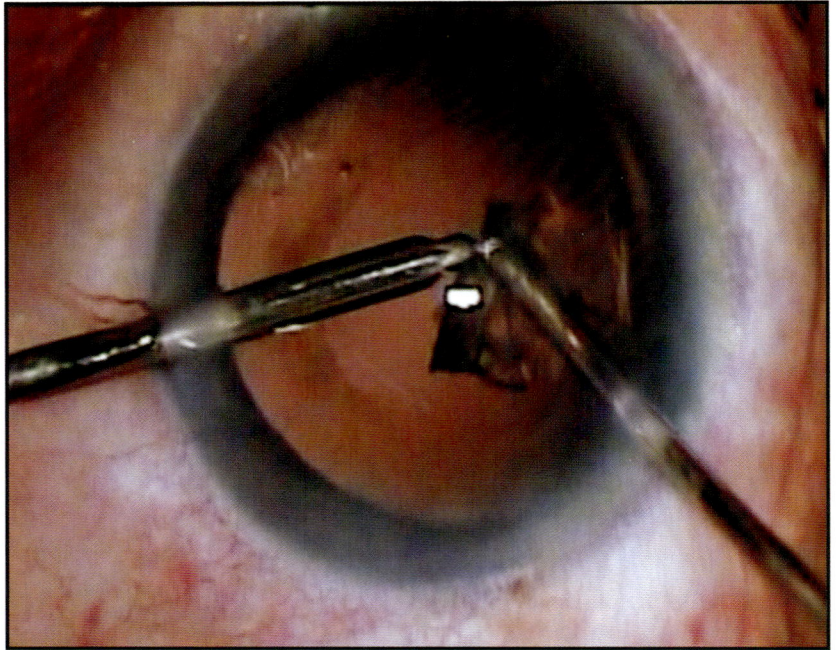

Fig. 14.2E: Cortical clean up with bimanual I and A

Capsular polishing: Instruments used:

- Simcoe
- Olive flap cannula
- Sandblast cannula
- Sandblast irrigation and aspiration cannula

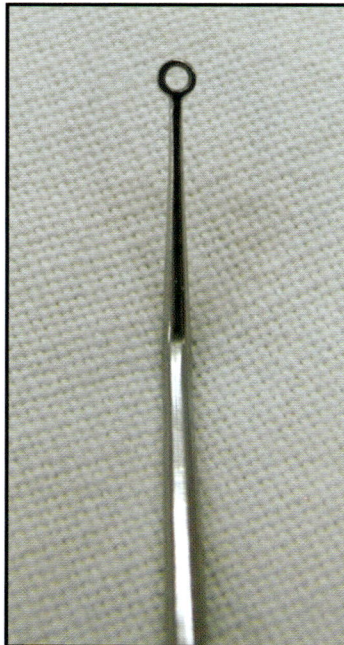

Fig. 14.3: Sandblast polisher for removal of PCO

15

Intraocular Lens

Ideal IOL: Should have the Following Characteristics

- Good optical property
- Non-antigenic and non-toxic
- Durable
- Easy to sterilize
- Optimal size to be implantable through the small incision
- Capable of being fabricated in the desired form.

Types of IOL

PCIOL
ACIOL
Scleral fixated IOL
Special: Aniridia lens—Central area of clear PMMA surrounded by an area of black color
Cosmetic IOL: IOL for cases of leukokoria
Surface coated IOL: Heparin coated IOL
Fluorine coated IOL

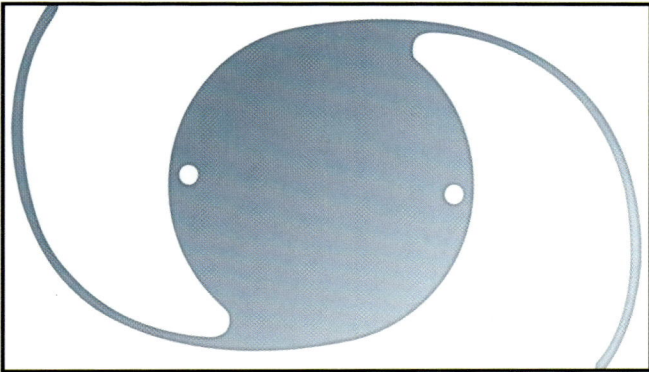

Fig. 15.1A: Single piece PMMA PCIOL

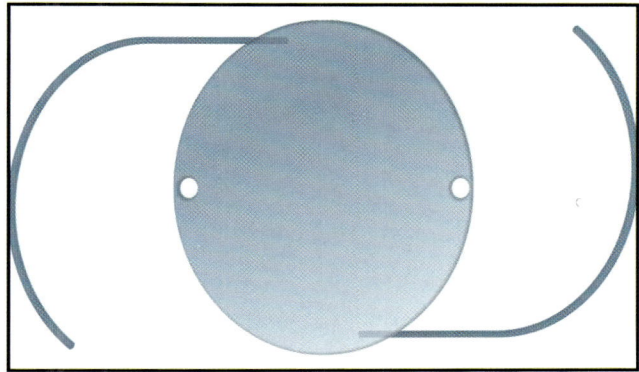

Fig. 15.1B: Three piece PMMA PCIOL

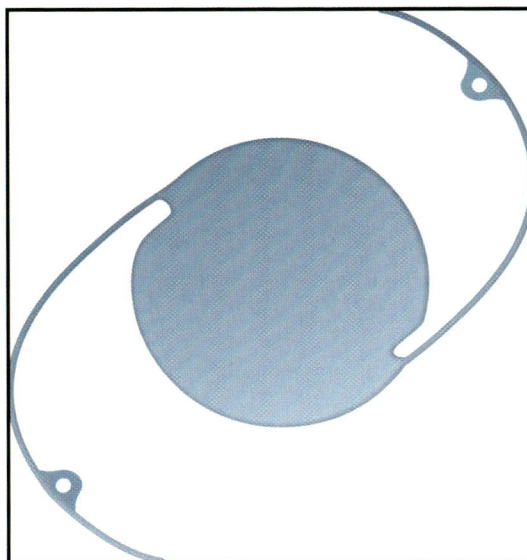

Fig. 15.1C: Scleral fixation IOL

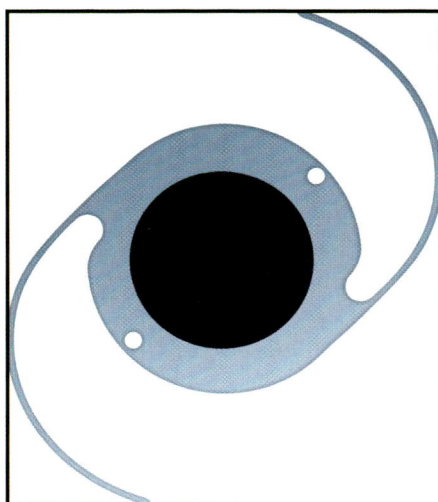

Fig. 15.1D: Cosmetic IOL

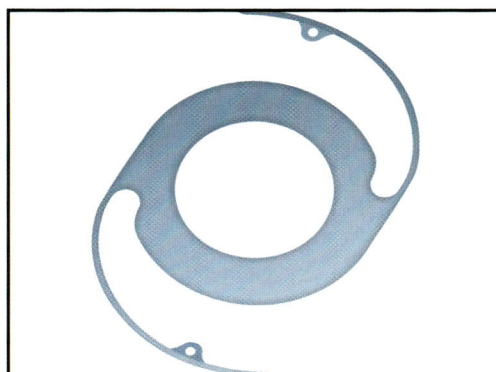

Fig. 15.1E: Aniridia IOL

PCIOL

Material—The Various Materials Used are

1. Rigid IOL–PMMA (Polymethyl methacrylate)
2. Foldable IOL–Silicone
3. Acrylic IOL—
   - Hydrophilic acrylic lens—Poly Hexa ethyl methacrylate hydrogels
   - Hydrophobic acrylic lens—Acrylate and methacrylate copolymers.

Size

5.25 mm × 12 mm
5.5 mm × 12 mm
6 mm × 12 mm
6 mm × 12.5 mm
6.5 mm × 13 mm

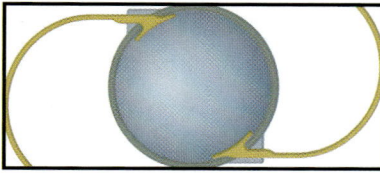

Fig. 15.2A: Foldable silicone IOL

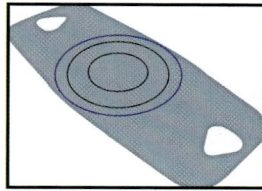

Fig. 15.2B: Rollable IOL

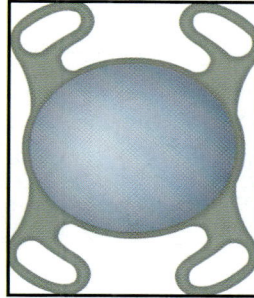

Fig. 15.2C: Hydrophillic IOL (Acreyos)

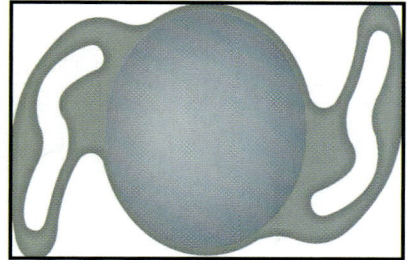

Fig. 15.2D: Hydrophillic foldable IOL (Acryfold)

ACIOL

Ideal ACIOL: Haptics with no closed loops
Peripherally wide, flat haptics
Flexible haptics.

Refractive property

- Unifocal
- Bifocal
- Multifocal :
  - Diffractive
  - Refractive
- Accommodative
- Toric
- Prolate

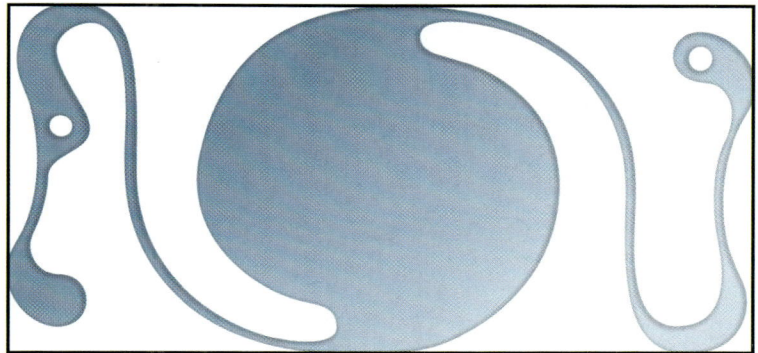

Fig. 15.3: ACIOL PMMA

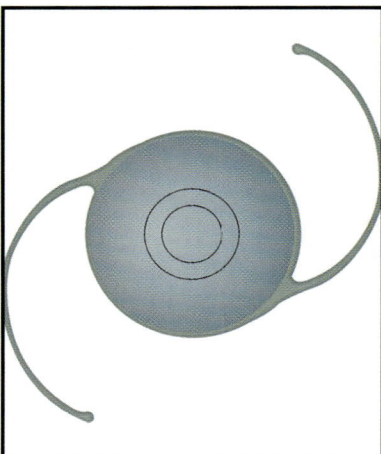

Fig. 15.4A: Bi focal PMMA IOL

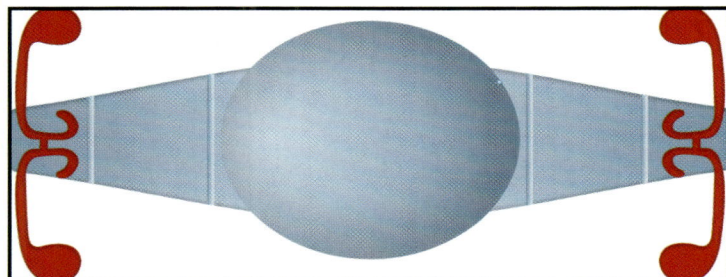

Fig. 15.4B: Accommodative IOL

Based on the number of pieces:

Single piece: Optic and haptic are made of the same material and has no joint. For example PMMA, acrylic IOL 3 pieces: Optic and Haptic are made of different material. For example, Acrysof IOL–Optic made of acrylic and haptic made of PMMA.

IOL material: A comparison

IOL material	Advantages	Disadvantages
PMMA	Low cost biocompatible	Requires large incision high incidence of PCO
Silicone foldable	Smaller incision low incidence of PCO	More decentration cannot be used in silicone filled eyes
Acrylic	Foldable low incidence of PCO filtration of blue light	Expensive

At present in rigid lenses PMMA lenses and in foldables hydrophobic acrylic lenses are ideal.

MULTIFOCAL IOL

The need for Multifocals:

To visualize, the distance, near and intermediate through the same lens or only one of these. Two or more images are formed at a time. The human brain works to ignore the out of focus image and accepts the clearest image. Hence the accommodation is in the brain and not in the eye. For this the brain takes some time to adapt.

Patients with multifocal implants are lesser dependant on spectacles as they see all the ranges of distance. However there is some compromise on quality (contrast) of the image.

The Principle:

- Refractive Multizonal design
- Diffractive design.

Refractive multizonal design: (Phenomenon of bending of light)

In this lens, multiple zones usually five will be there for near, intermediate and distance. Each zone is meant for a particular distance. Refractive multifocal IOL is dependant on the size of the pupil and the light distribution is unequal. The light distribution is in the ratio of 50:13:37 for distance, intermediate and near respectively. For example–Array's lens

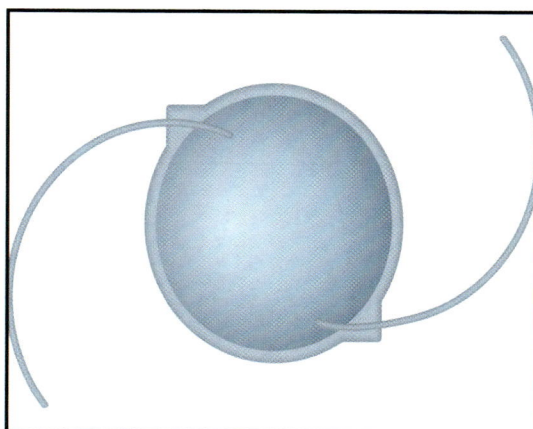

Fig. 15.5A: Mulifocal IOL (Array's)

Diffractive design: (Phenomenon of spreading of light)

In this there are two points of focus. The first focus is at the interphase of diffraction and the other focus is at the base power of the lens. Diffractive are independent of the pupil size and the light distribution is equal for both distance and near.

Prerequisites for Multifocal IOL:

- Accurate biometry
- Meticulous surgical technique
- In the bag, well centered IOL
- Minimal induced astigmatism
- Proper patient selection
- Preoperative patient counseling.

Contraindications:

- Posterior segment pathology
- Fundus pathology warranting future LASER therapy
- Astigmatism more than 1 diopter
- Extremes of refractive errors
- Very young or very old patients
- Dislocated or subluxated lens
- Previous ocular surgery.

Indications for Multifocal IOL:

- Young patients with cataract
- Presbyopic patients (PREFLEX)
- Refractive lens exchange patients (REFLEX).

Examples for Multifocal IOL

- ARRAY is refractive multifocal
- Technis ZM 900 is diffractive multifocal
- Rezoom has balance optics and has a combination of both refractive and diffractive optical properties
- Restor.

Multifocal IOLs are a good alternative to monofocal but only in carefully selected patients. They demand accurate biometry and meticulous surgery.

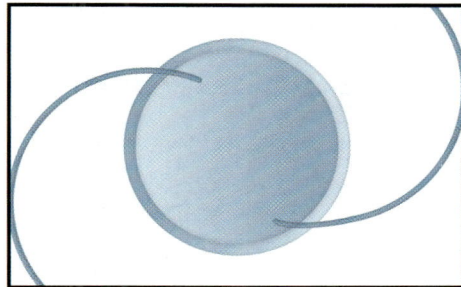

Fig. 15.5B: Rezoom lens

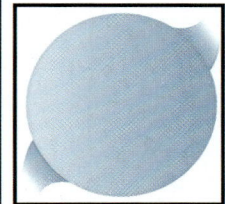

Fig. 15.5C: Restor lens

16

Wound Closure

In SICS, most of the times the wound is self sealing due to the valvular effect of the tunnel. At the end of surgery, the anterior chamber is deepened by injecting saline or BSS through the side port entry and the integrity of the wound is checked by pressing the area near the limbus. The side port wound is sealed by hydrating the stromal layers of the cornea by injecting fluid into the stromal layers of the external lip of the side port wound.

The conjunctival flap is pulled over to the sclerocorneal incision and minimal cautery is applied to seal the edges.

Suturing the wound may be essential in certain conditions

1. Scleral tunnel more than 6.5 mm in length.
2. If there is a leaking tunnel.
3. Premature entry.
4. In pediatric cases where the scleral wall is thin.

SUTURES

Sutures Can be

• **Vertical Sutures**

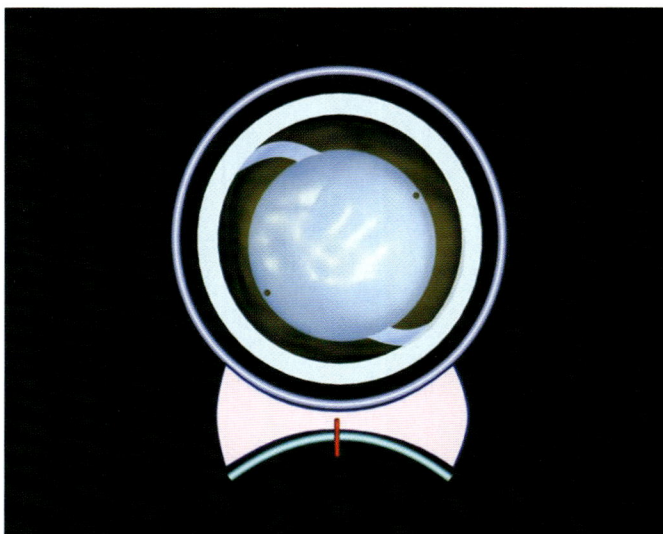

Fig. 16.1A: Vertical simple suture

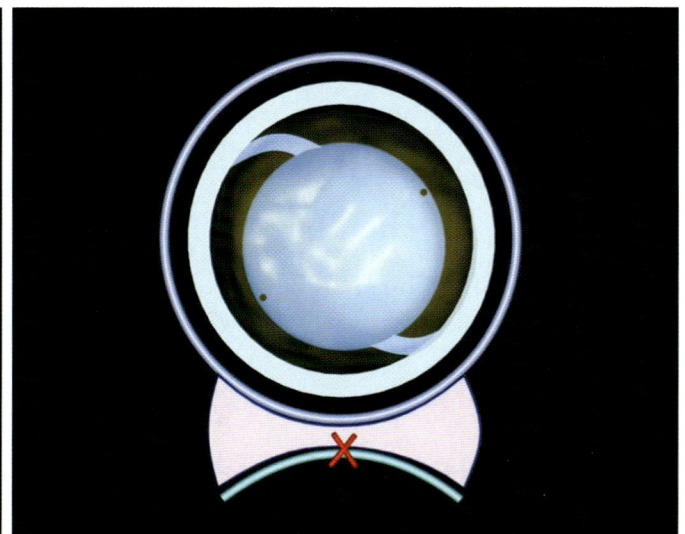

Fig. 16.1B: vertical cross suture

• Horizontal Sutures

1. Shepherd's single horizontal

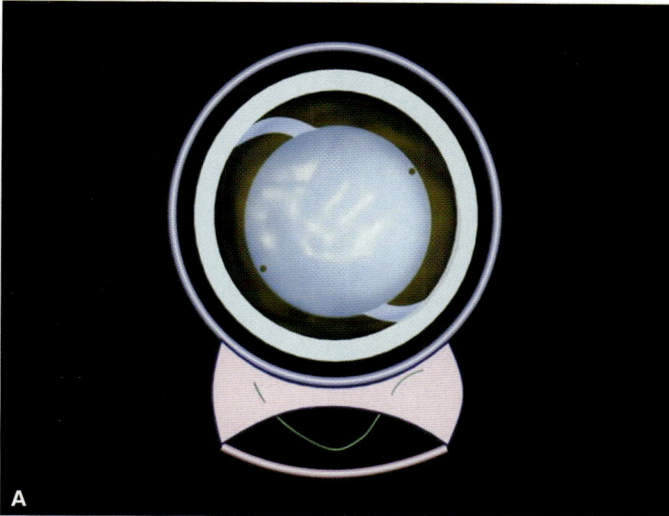

Step 1

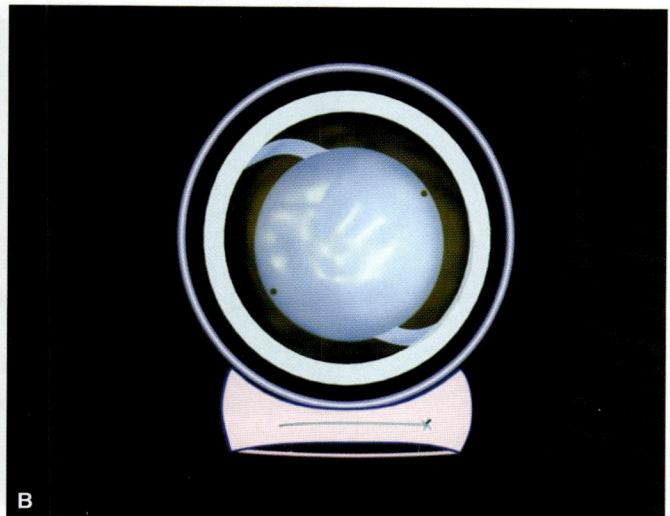

Step 2

Figs 16.2A and B: Shepherd's horizontal suture

2. Fine's infinity suture

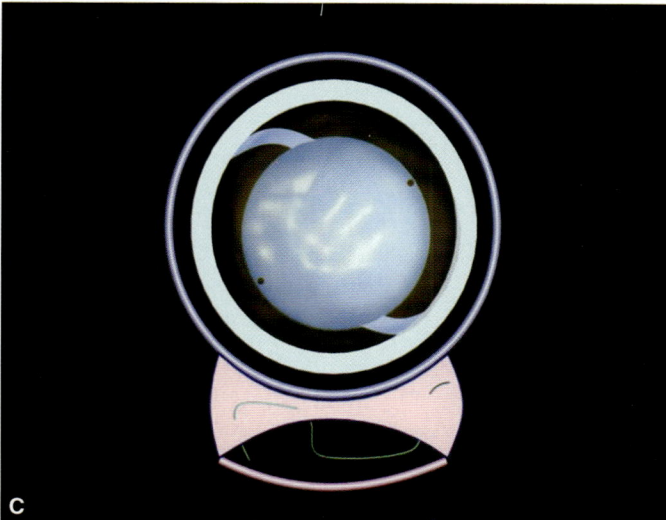

Step 1

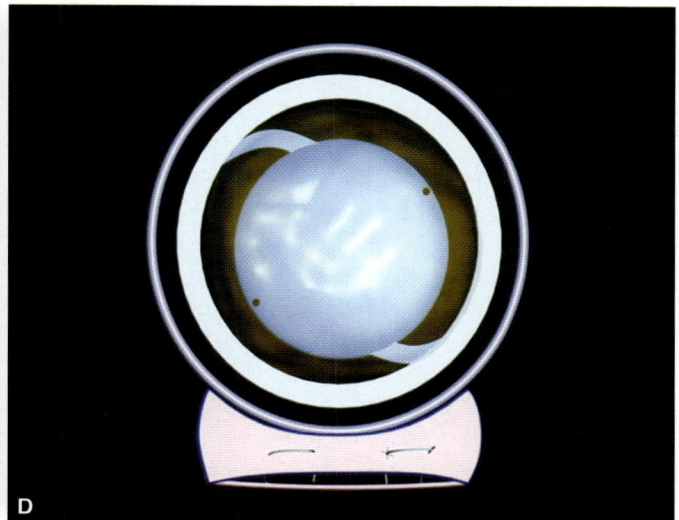

Step 2

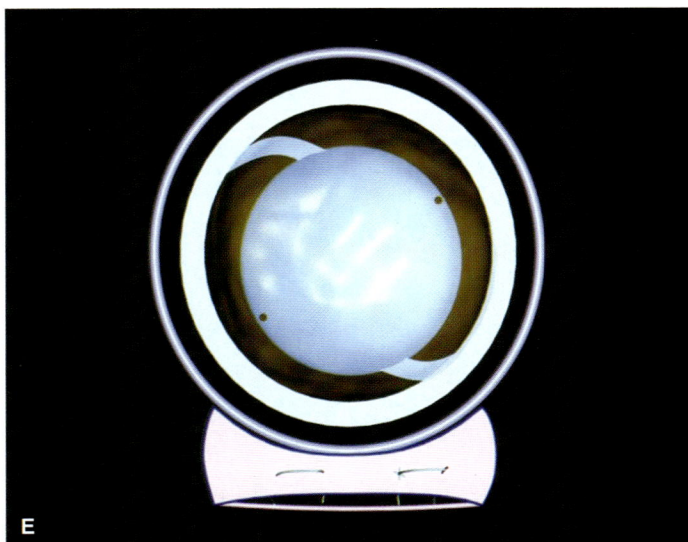

Step 3

Figs 16.2C to E: Fine's infinity suture

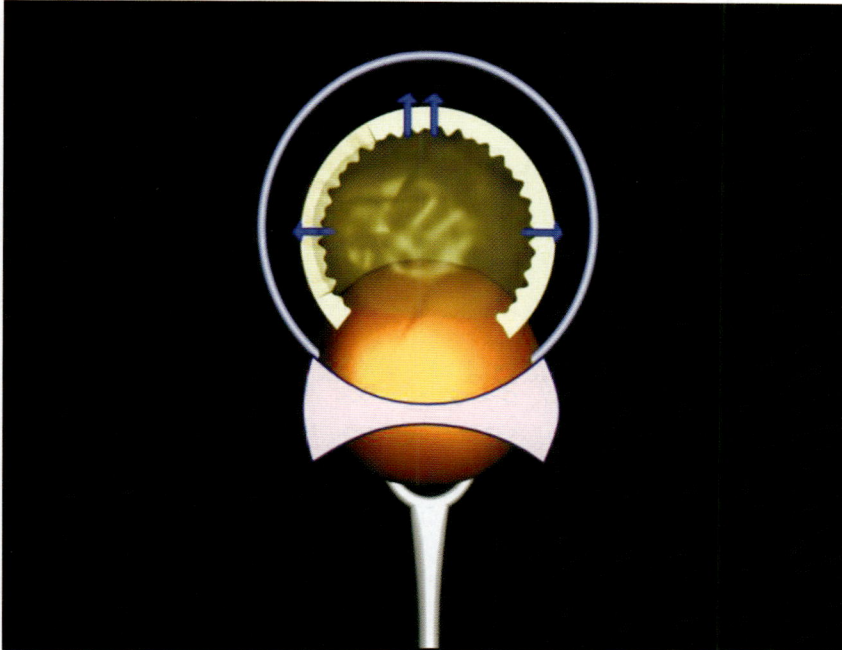

SICS

Conversion to

PHACO

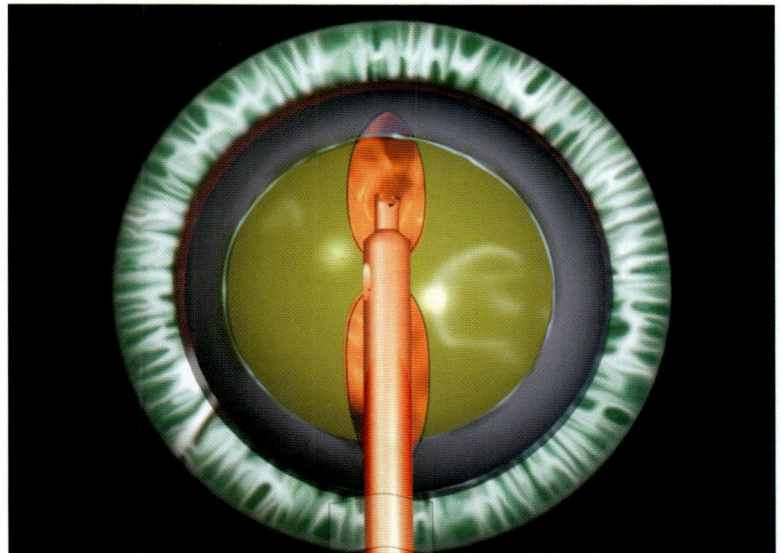

17

Conversion to Phaco

STEPS

Most of the steps in SICS and phacoemulsification are common exceptions being the nuclear management. The following steps are easier in phacoemulsification for surgeons who have mastered SICS:

Incision: A small and a clear corneal incision is easier and faster to make than a sclerocorneal tunnel.

Rhexis: Making a small rhexis is easier than a wide rhexis.

Hydroprocedures: Minimal hydrodissection, of the times only hydrodelineation is sufficient.

Cortical aspiration: Automated bimanual cortical aspiration is easier than manual cortical aspiration.

Pupillary dilatation is well maintained in phaco compared to SICS.

Phaco IOL size is smaller than that of SICS IOL hence insertion into the bag is easy.

Difficulties

1. Understanding the mechanics of the machine.

2. Management of the nucleus with the machine for beginners.

3. Injury to the cornea, capsule and iris due to phacoemulsification surgery.

How to Proceed?

1. A good knowledge of the machine and its mechanics is essential.

2. Mastering the technique of rhexis in all types of cataracts. Use of capsular staining dyes will be helpful in this step.

3. Hydroprocedures and nuclear rotation technique should be mastered.

4. During nuclear management phaco energy is utilized depending on hardness of nucleus, e.g. linear mode, pulse mode or burst mode.

5. Liberal usage of viscoelastics to maintain the anterior chamber and avoid damage to corneal endothelium.

6. Finally the surgeon should develop a good hand and feet co-ordination in operating the machine, where he needs to use simultaneously both eyes, hands, legs and ears.

7. As and when the phaco surgeon is not comfortable with phaco procedure, it is ideal to convert phaco into SICS at any stage of surgery.

Section
3

Phacoemulsification

18 Do You Know Your Machine?

Knowledge of the phaco machine is half of the phaco procedure. Using a machine without proper knowledge is like providing a knife to a child as a toy.

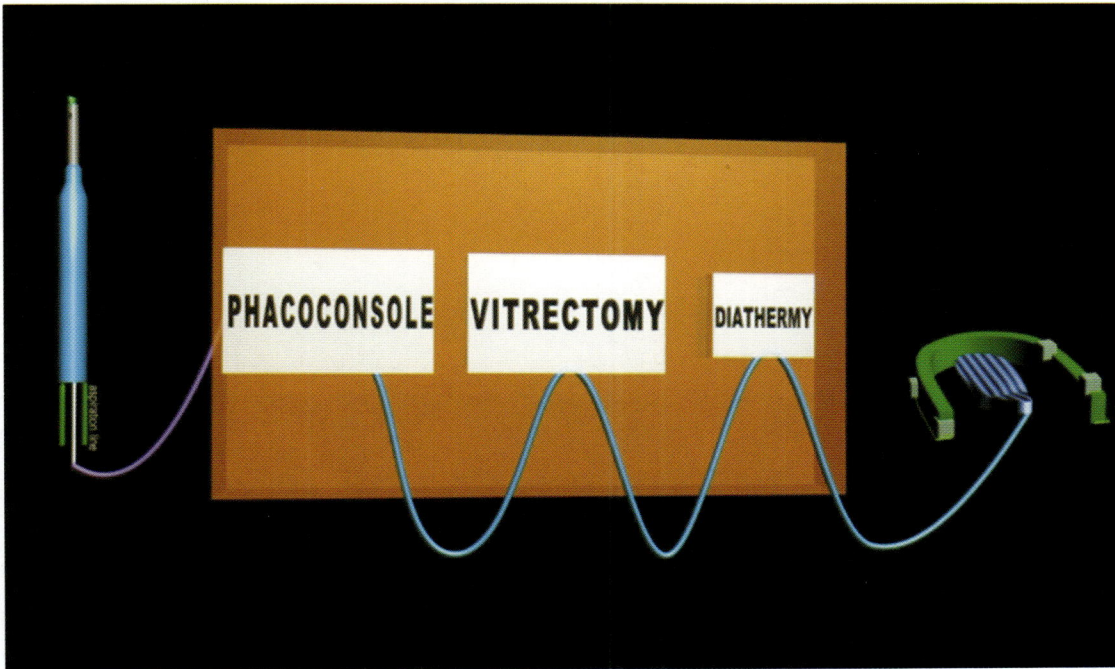

Fig. 18.1: Phaco machine, probe, console and foot pedal

HAND PIECE

The handpiece converts electrical energy into mechanical vibrations at ultrasonic speed (47 KHz). It consists of

1. Detachable titanium tip

   There are various types of tips depending on the configuration of bevel– 0°, 15°, 30°, 45°, 60°.

   0° and 15° have maximum holding capacity.

   45° and 60° have maximum cutting capacity.

   Hence in phaco I (trenching and sculpting) we use 45° tip.

   For holding the fragment, in phaco II we use 0 and 15° tip

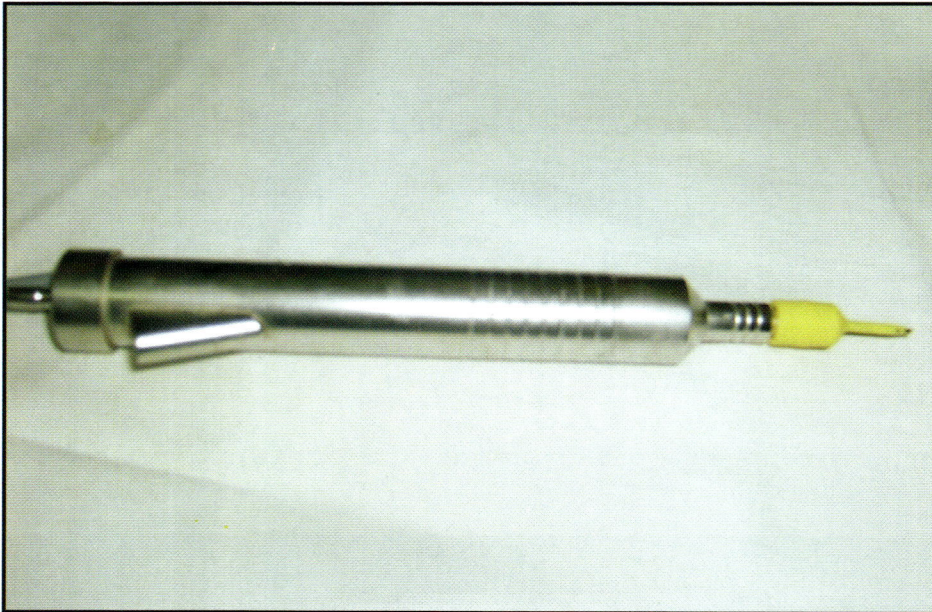

Fig. 18.2A: Phaco hand piece

For classical phaco the author
advises
Phaco I – 30°/45°
phaco II – 0°/30°
Stop and chop – 15°
Direct chop – 0°

2. Depending on the configuration of the shaft

   (a) Cobra tip

   (b) Kelman tip

   (c) Flat head tip

   (d) Square tip

   (e) Scalpel tip

   (f) Microflow tip

   (g) Diaphragmatic tip

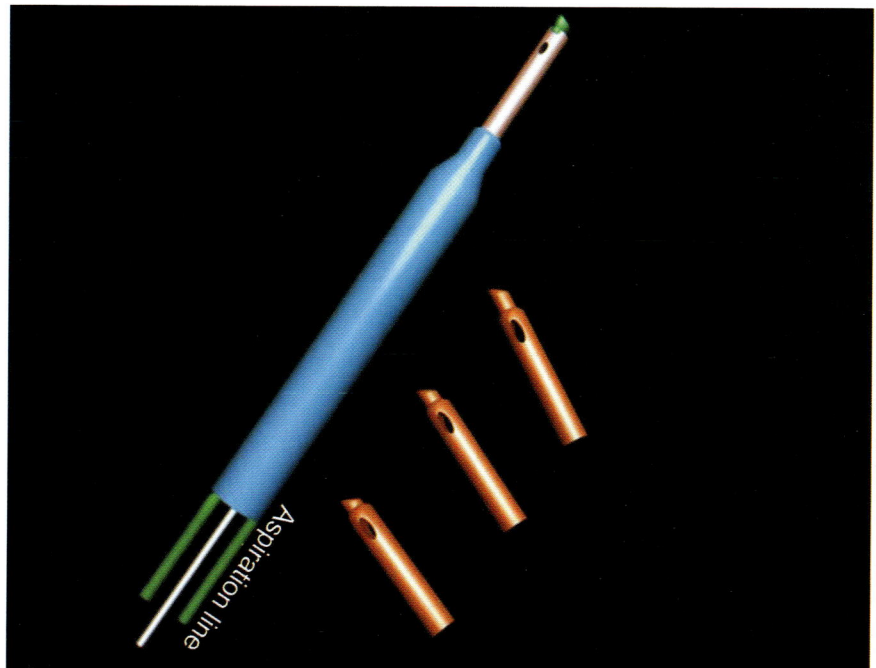

Fig. 18.2B: Phaco hand piece and tips 15°, 30° and 45°

| Cobra tip | ABS tip | Microflow tip |

| Mackool tip | Kelman tip |

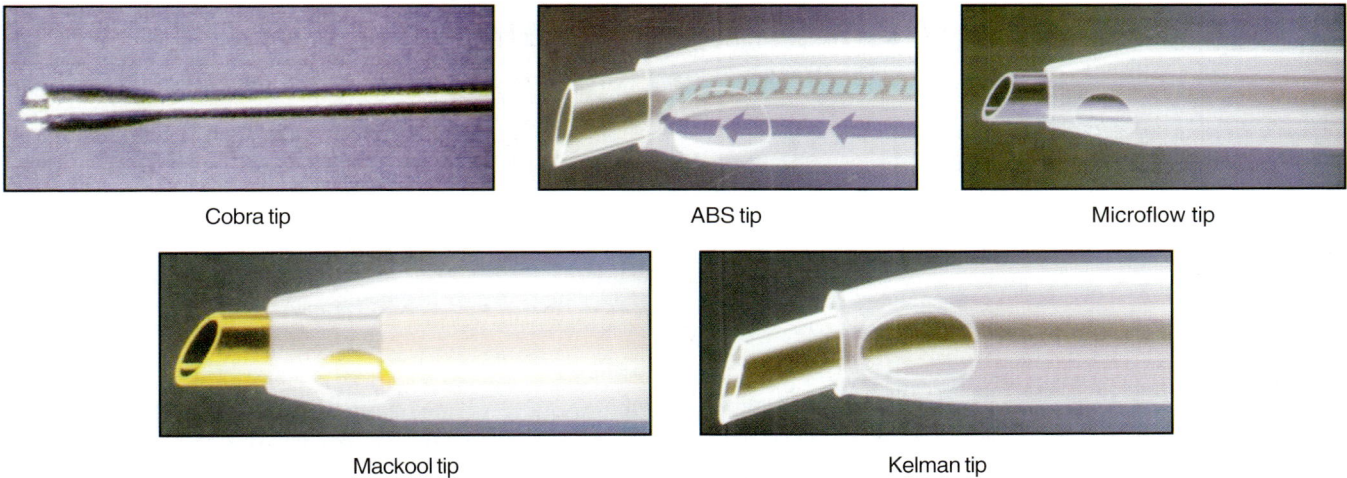

Fig. 18.3: Phaco tips

- Microflow tip has external ribs. It increases the cooling capacity.
- Cobra tip has increased surface of ultrasound origin thus reduces level of energy required.
- Kelman tip has 30° angulation and the cavitational effect is transmitted to the lens instead of endothelium.
- *Diaphragmatic tip:* In this we can use high vacuum levels with no risk of surge.

PRECAUTION

While using the second instrument care should be taken to avoid contact of second instrument to the phaco tip, which will damage the tip reducing the sharpness.

Sleeves

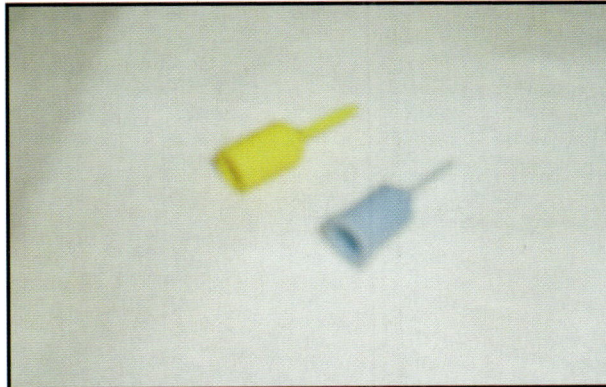

Fig. 18.4: Sleeves

Made up of silicon

Two types are there :

(a) Single walled

(b) Double walled

Double wall has the advantage of reducing the heat energy transmission from the tip to the wound. Hence reduces thermal burns and maintains flow even in narrow incision.

Adjustment: It is preferable to adjust the sleeve exposing the titanium tip of 1mm. If there are air bubbles in the procedure adjustment of the sleeve will reduce the bubbles.

MECHANISM OF ULTRASOUND HANDPIECE

a) Jack hammer effect - Direct mechanical effect due to axial vibration of tip.

b) Cavitational effect - Movement of the tip at ultrasonic frequency creates areas of high and low pressure. The dissolved gases become bubbles which explode releasing energy.

c) Acoustic breakdown by ultrasonic shock waves.

Console

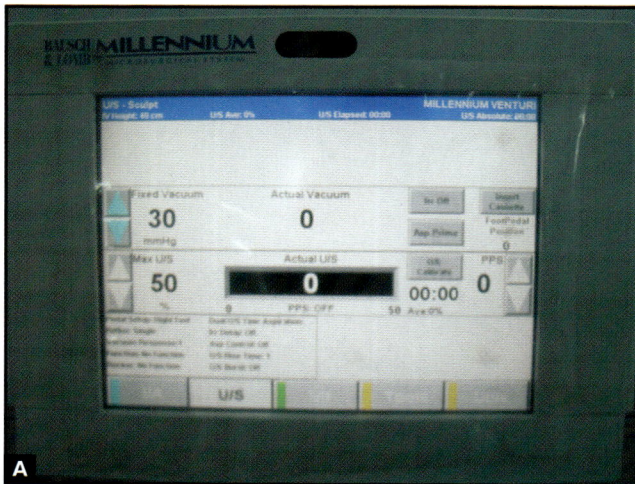

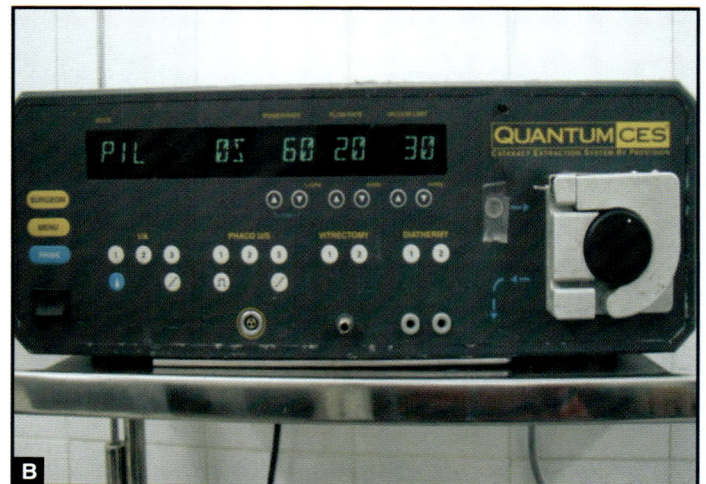

Figs 18.5A and B: Consoles (A) Millenium machine (B) Quantum machine

Console consists of the following subunits

a) Pump console which creates vacuum

b) Ultrasound console for producing ultrasonic energy

c) Vitrectomy console for anterior vitrectomy

d) Cautery console for coagulating bleeders

Pumps

Pumps are of two types:

1) Peristaltic pump

2) Venturi pump

1. Peristaltic Pump

This pump has multiple rollers which compress the tube and draw the fluid from the eye. Occlusion of the tube by solids creates vacuum.

There are two terms to be understood

1) Flow rate
2) Vacuum

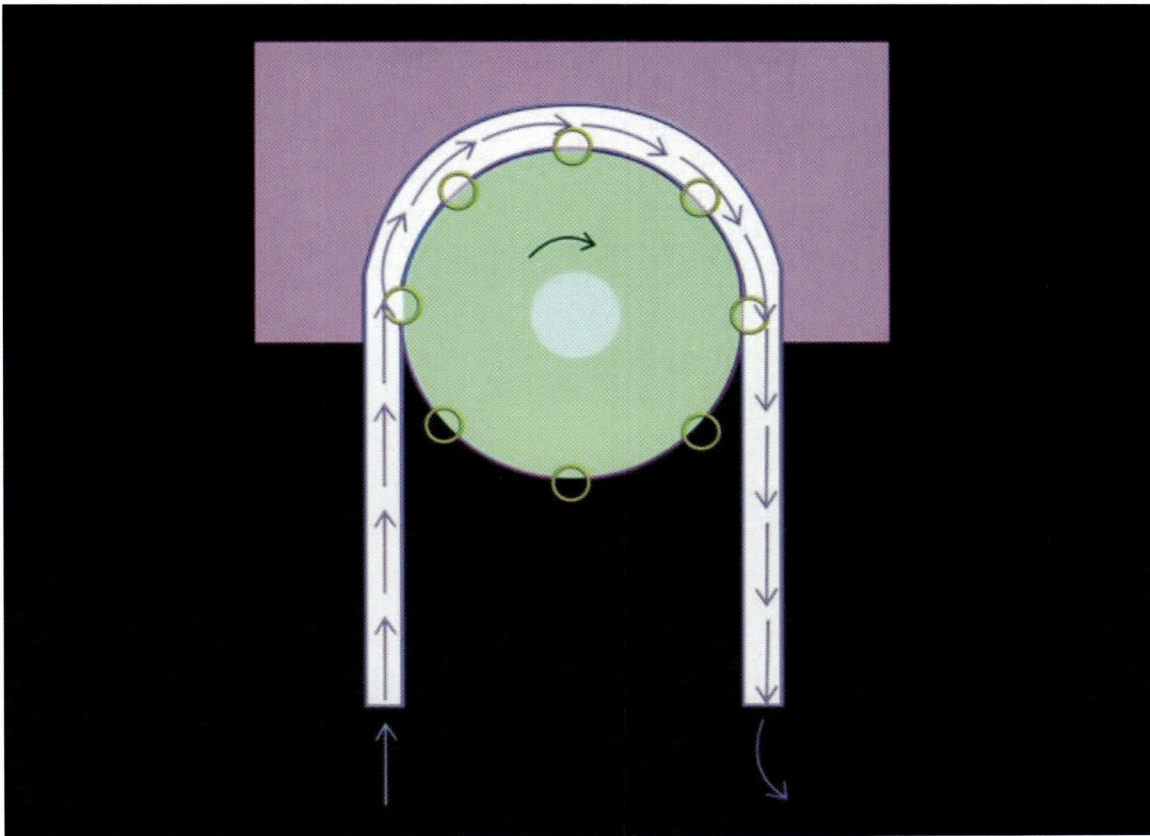

Fig. 18.6A: Peristaltic pump

Flow rate

It indicates the amount of fluid drawn from the eye into the pump so the correct term is Aspiration Flow Rate (AFR).

It is directly proportional to the pump speed.

If the aspiration flow rate is high it automatically draws more fluid from the bottle as indicated in the drip chamber. It mirrors the intensity of the current in the anterior chamber. If the pump flow is high the rise time decreases.

Vacuum

It depends on the rotational speed of the pump and occlusion.

Flow rate is independent of occlusion

At low flow rate there is no vacuum without occlusion

At high flow rate vacuum is created even with out occlusion due to the resistance offered by small opening of the tip. Hence at high flow rates peristaltic pump acts as venturi pump.

The author advises that the beginners should always start the procedure using the peristaltic pump.

2. Venturi Pump

Compressed Air (using the electrical compressor) or nitrogen (using cylinders) is directed through a chamber which creates vacuum. This aspirates fluid which gets collected in cassettes. Hence frequent emptying of the cassettes is essential. The vacuum created is independent of occlusion and the rise time (of vacuum) is faster than the peristaltic pump. The flow rate and vacuum cannot be adjusted separately. They proportionately increase or decrease.

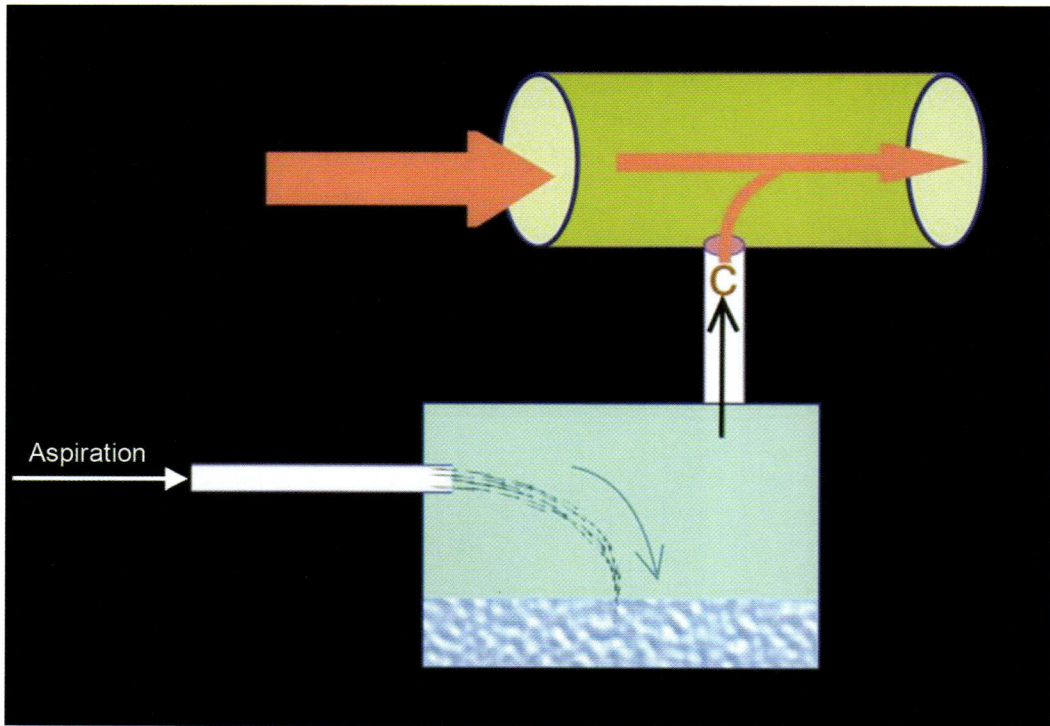

Fig .18.6B: Venturi pump

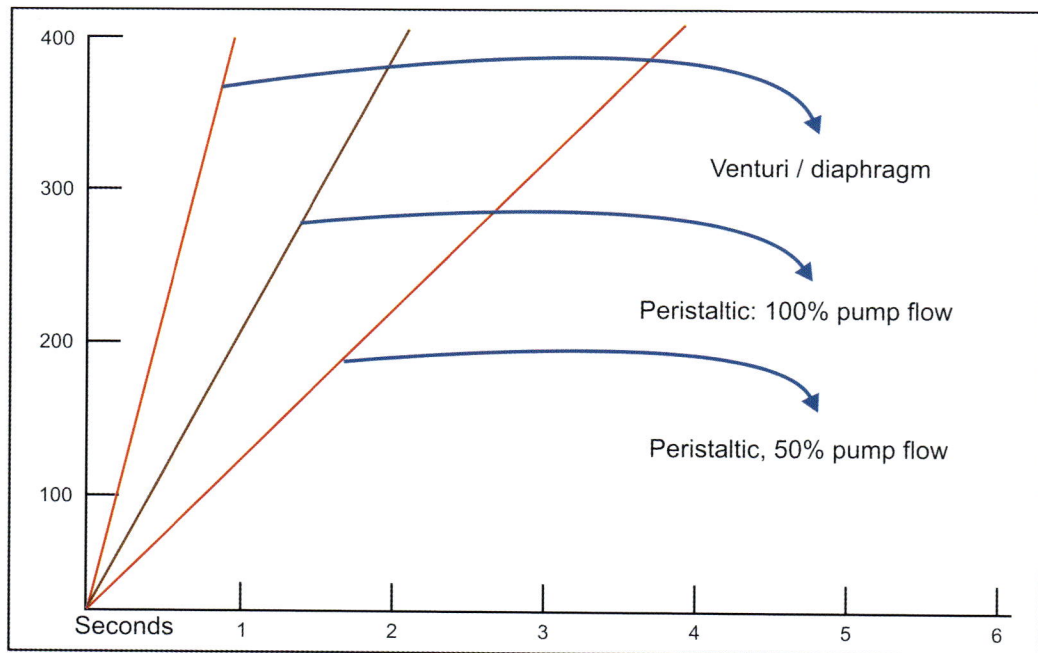

Fig. 18.7: Graph showing rise time

Rise time: It is a measure of how soon the vacuum builds up to the preset value when the flow is restricted.

19

Phacodynamics

A good fluid balance should be maintained

INFLOW

Is the fluid entering the eye. It depends on the

1) Height of the bottle
2) Diameter of the tube
3) Pressure in the bottle
4) Resistance offered at the incision and the opening of the tube

Inflow can be increased by adjusting the height of the bottle manually or mechanically (modern machines have the facility to adjust the height of the bottle by foot switch).

If the flow is insufficient, the diameter of the tube can be altered by using blood transfusion sets or using the second bottle which is connected by TUR (Transurethral resections) tube.

Positive pressure in the bottle can be created using air pump or a fish pump.

Resistance offered at the incision

A narrow and long tunnel causes collapse of the sleeve. Hence it reduces the inflow. This can be overcome by correct size incision and double walled sleeves. Another way of increasing inflow is by using AC maintainers.

OUTFLOW

Depends on:

1. Vacuum
2. Flow rate
3. Wound leak

Whenever there is a collapse of the anterior chamber the outflow is reduced by decreasing the vacuum and the flow rate.

Wound Leak

Can be due to:

1. Incorrect sized keratome
2. Incorrect sized side entry
3. Incorrect sized phaco tip or choppers
4. Improper incision.

Whenever there is wound leak, convert into non-phacotechnique or close the wound. Take a fresh incision. (e.g. superior incision can be closed, and restarted with temporal incision).

SURGE AND VENTING

Surge means anterior chamber collapse
Venting is prevention of surge.

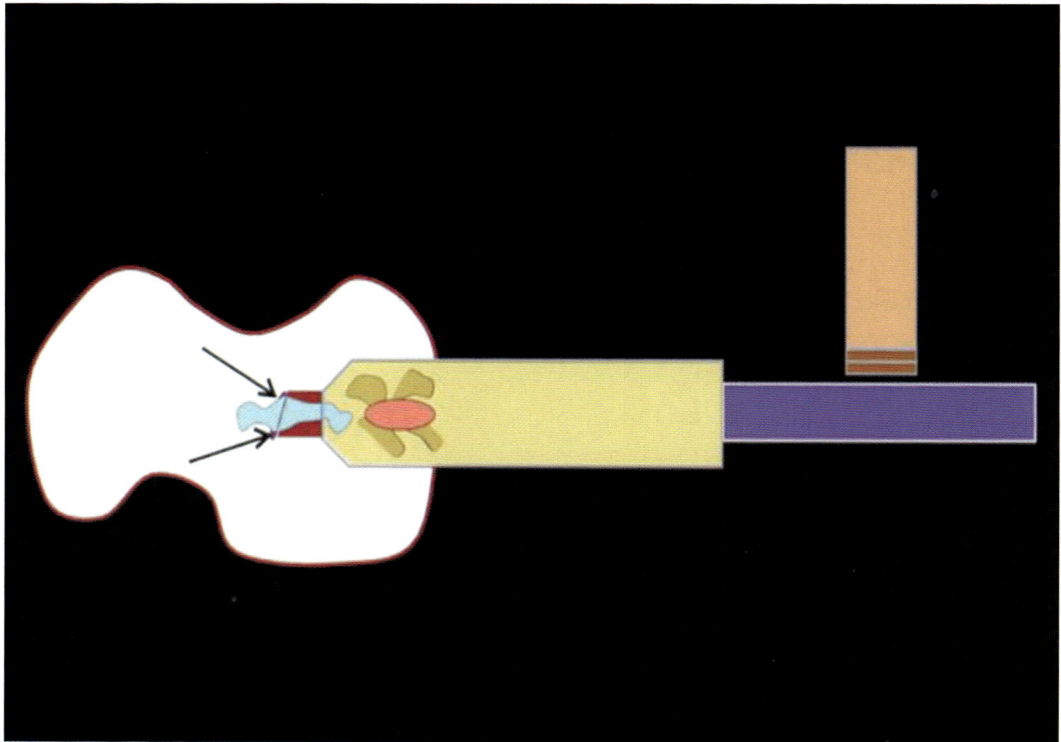

Fig. 19.1: Mechanism of surge; sudden release of obstruction creates an anterior chamber collapse

When we occlude the tip with nuclear fragment high vacuum is created in the tubing. When occlusion is broken, at the tip, the high-pressured fluid from the anterior chamber is pushed into the aspiration line resulting in sudden collapse of the anterior chamber. This phenomenon is known as surge. Surge causes damage to the corneal endothelium and lens capsule due to the mechanical touch of the phaco tip.

To prevent surge the machines are having protective mechanism called venting.

Venting is of two types:

1) Air venting

2) Fluid venting

The phenomenon of venting is by creating a leak in the aspiration line. This leak is created by the valvular mechanism, which is controlled by a microprocessor (sensor) which is connected between the phaco tip and the pump.

Whenever there is sudden change in the pressure the vent valve opens. This is with the help of a sensor. When there is opening of the valve, air or fluid enters the aspiration line resulting in the low pressure in the aspiration line and preventing the surge (anterior chamber collapse)

Air enters the system and breaks the vacuum.

In air venting, air enters into the system by an opening vent valve.

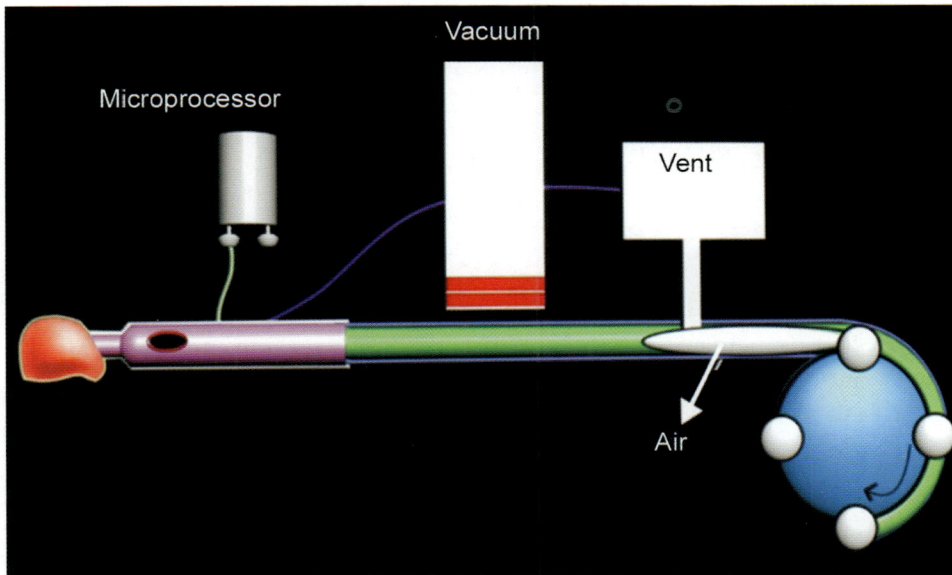

Fig. 19.2A: Air venting

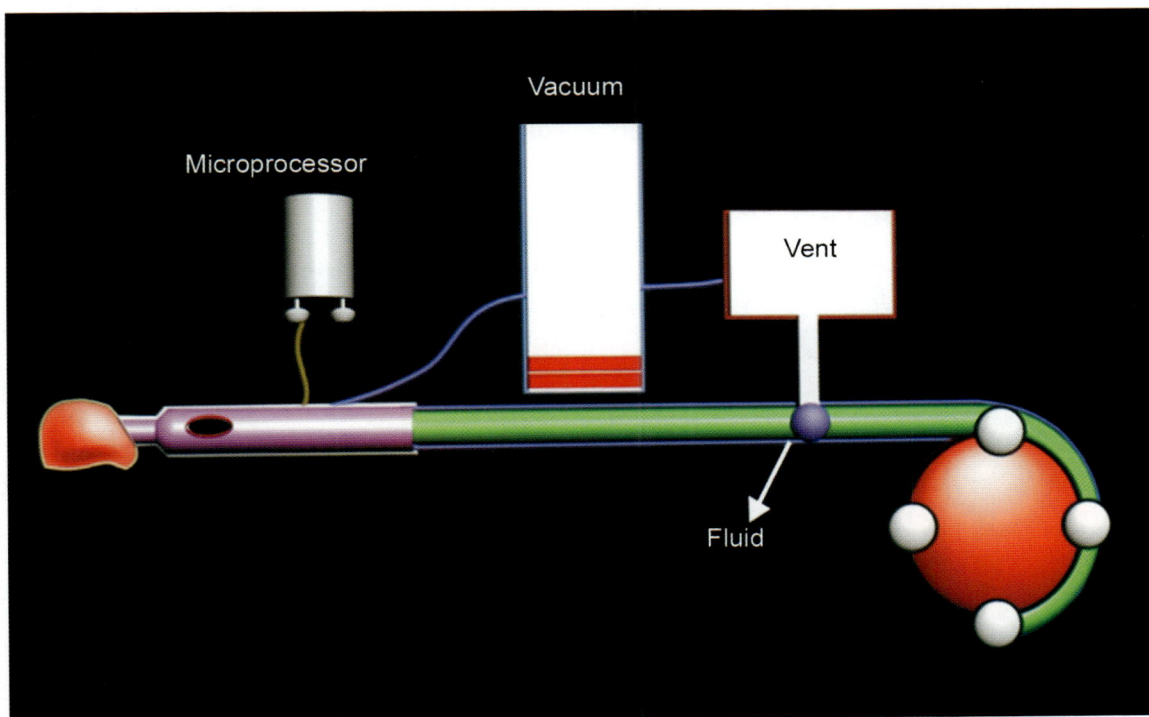

Fig. 19.2B: Fluid venting. Fluid enters the system and breaks the vacuum

In fluid venting, fluid enters the system from the infusion bottle.

Surge can also be prevented by careful operation of foot pedal.

Surge is minimal with higher end machines, which are incorporated with the sensor (microprocessor), which can detect the slightest change in the pressure in the aspiration line.

Peristaltic Pump: Relation between the foot pedal position, time, aspiration flow rate (AFR), to produce vacuum.

Table 19.1: Relation between time, AFR and Vacuum

Footpedal	Time	AFR	Vacuum
Position	0.1 Sec	20 cc/ Min	Minimum
Full	2.0 Sec	20 cc/Min	50%
Full	4.0 Sec	20 cc / Min	100%
Half	2.0 Sec	40 cc/ Min	50%
Full	2.0 Sec	40 cc/Min	100%

Surge can be controlled by using foot pedal position or by decreasing the AFR.

Whenever more vacuum is needed, increase the AFR or wait until you reach the maximum vacuum (rise time) in full foot pedal position.

VENTURI PUMP

Table 19.2: Relation between foot pedal position and time to produce vacuum

Foot Pedal	Time	Vacuum
50%	0.25 Sec	100 mm Hg
50%	0.50 Sec	200 mm Hg
100%	1.0 Sec	400 mm Hg (Full)

It is to be noted that vacuum control is mainly on the foot pedal and there is no aspiration flow rate adjustment.

Bottle Height Versus Flow

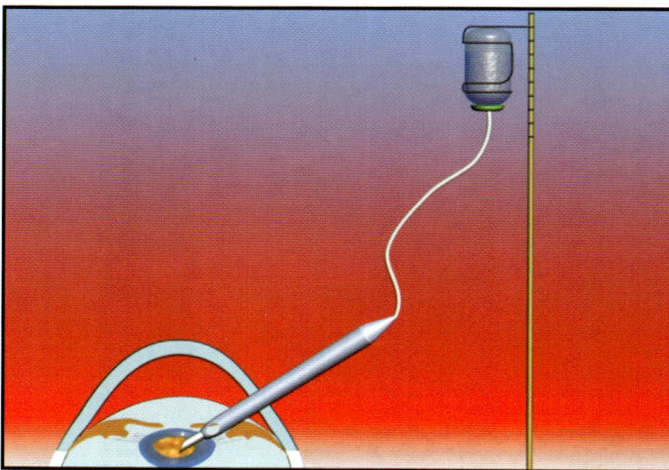

Fig. 19.3A: Note that if the bottle height is increased AC becomes deep, hence appropriate height of bottle should be maintained

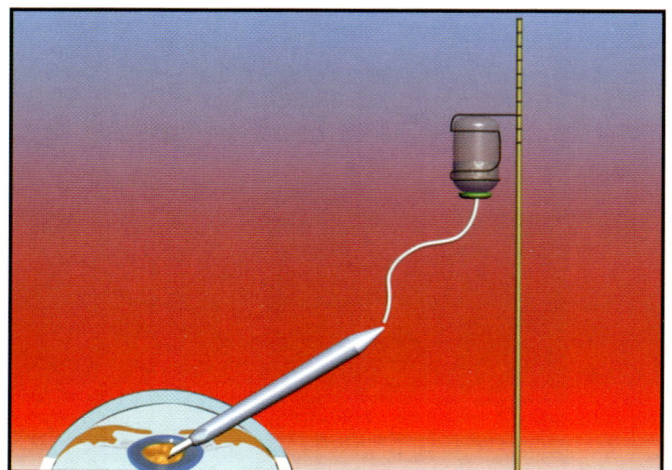

Fig. 19.3B: When bottle height is decreased AC becomes shallow

If we increase the bottle height the flow will not increase in peristaltic machine due to resistance by the pump rollers. In venturi machine the flow increases, as there is no resistance of the pump.

PHACO POWER

Full Power = 100%

The energy delivered at the tip depends upon the amount of time the foot pedal is kept depressed in position 3(phaco time) and the amount of average phaco power used.

Absolute phaco time (APT) = phaco time × average phaco power

APT will be less when phaco time and phaco power are less.

The lower the APT the lesser will be the corneal damage.

Adverse effects of more energy are:

  i. Corneal endothelial damage
 ii. Piercing of the nucleus
iii. Damage to the capsule
 iv. Damage to the iris
  v. Corneal incisional burns.

PHACO 1

SCULPT – TRENCH

Use Appropriate Power

- Tip engagement
    1) 1/3 tip engaged
    2) 2/3 tip engaged
    3) full tip engaged
- Power adjustment 10 to 70%
- Linear velocity of phaco needle.

SCULPTING

Change of the foot pedal position depending on the density of the nucleus (linear phaco).

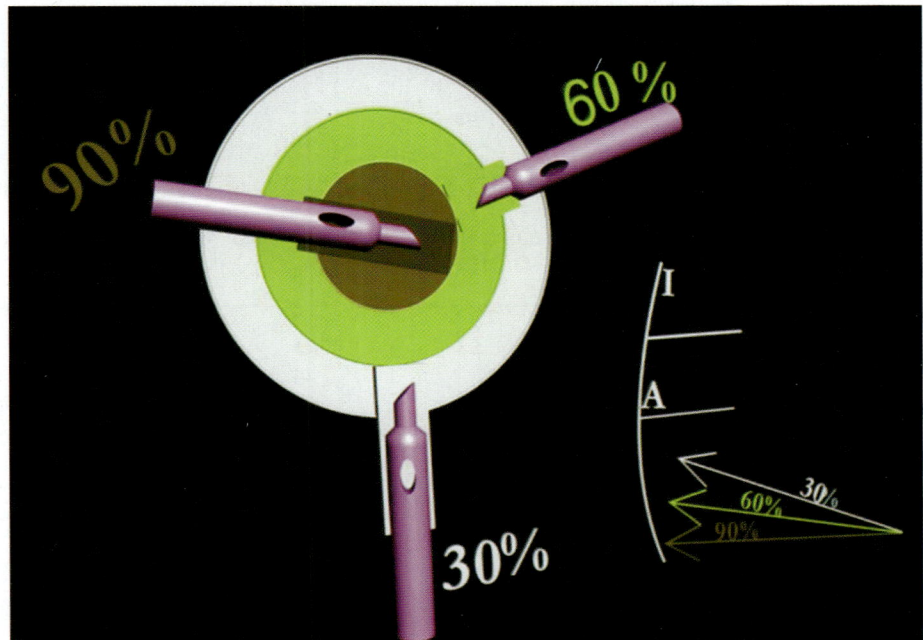

Fig. 19.4A: Phaco power should be used appropriately as shown, for central core of nucleus upto 90%

Individual Machine Characteristics

Same parameters may not hold good for all machines. One must be familiar with all the features given in the machine to maximize the results.

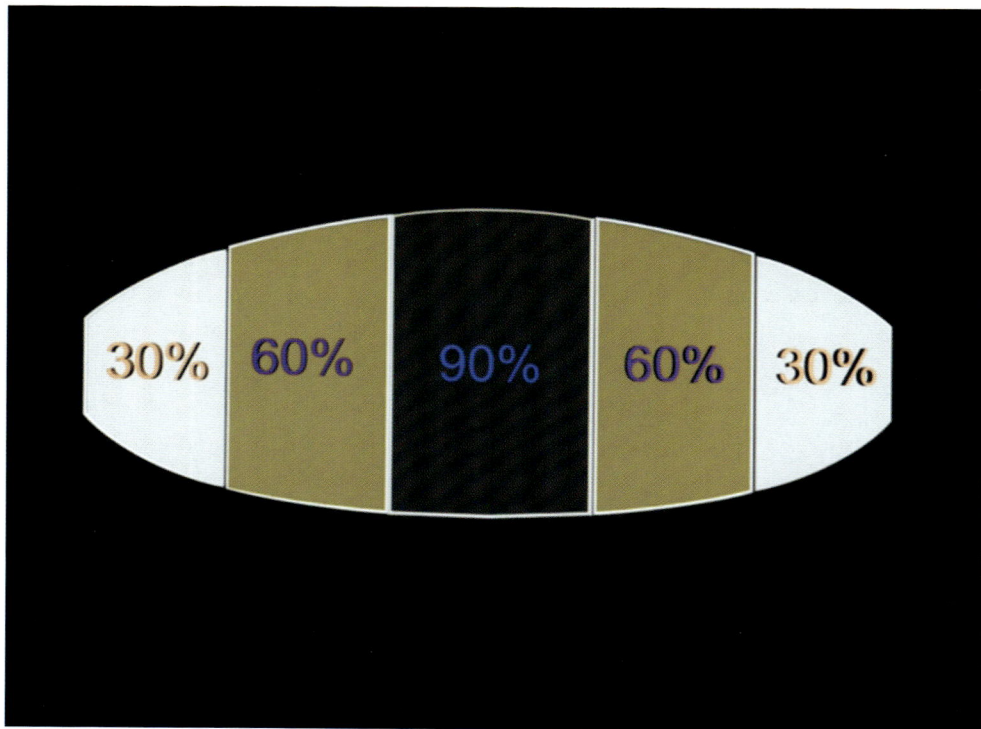

Fig. 19.4B: Appropriate power has to be used when dealing with central nucleus(90%), mid peripheral nucleus (60%), peripheral nucleus (30%)

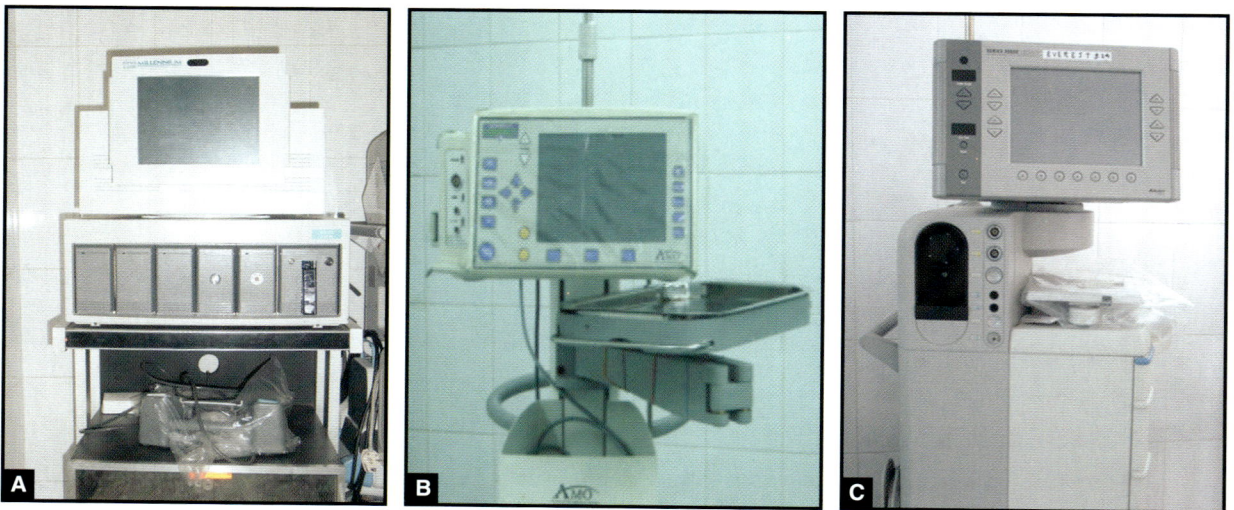

Figs 19.5A to C: Phacomachines, A. Millenium, Bausch and Lomb, B. AMO Sovereign, C. Legacy machine

One must be familiar with the tones provided to each mode.

Linear mode, pulse mode, burst mode, hyper pulse mode, I/A mode and occlusion mode so that we can adjust the aspiration rate and foot pedal position.

Linear mode: In this mode continuous steady phaco energy is delivered. It is proportionate to the position of the foot pedal. In the initial stage of foot pedal 10% of energy is delivered. As we depress the pedal the energy goes on increasing to the maximum preset level. This is useful in the initial sculpting and trenching. Depending on the hardness of the nucleus the foot pedal should be pressed sufficiently.

Pulse Mode

In this mode the energy is delivered at regular intervals (pulses), "ON and "OFF" for an equal period of time and it will be increasing steadily depending on the position of the foot pedal. By delivering energy at regular intervals the power delivered is reduced to half and produces some cooling effect on the tip.

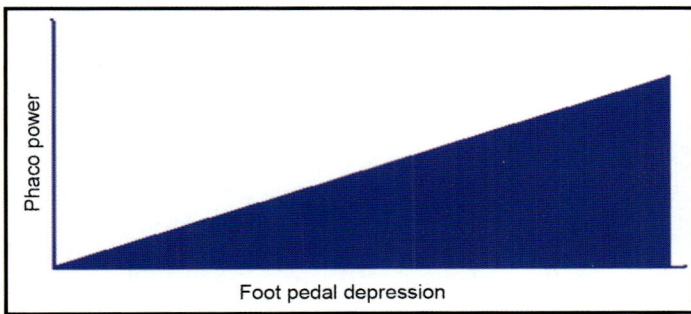

Fig. 19.6A: Linear mode—the energy released will be proportionate to the foot pedal position

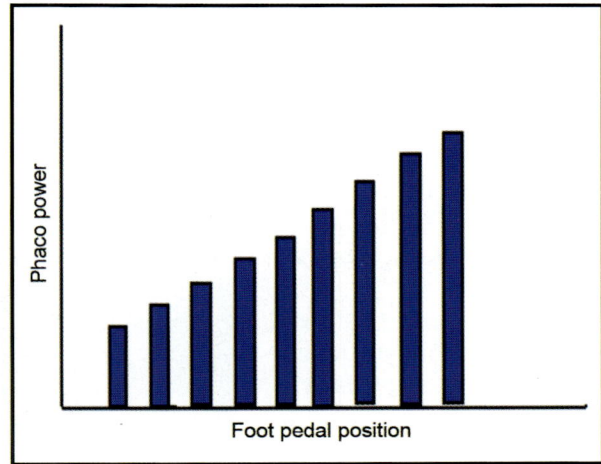

Fig. 19.6B: Pulse mode—the energy delivered will be at regular intervals and as the foot pedal is depressed the phaco power will increase

Burst Mode

In this mode the preset energy is delivered even at the initial step of the foot pedal and during every pulse and the energy is delivered at regular intervals as in the pulse mode. As we depress the footpedal further the frequency of the pulses increases. It is useful in dealing with hard cataracts and to hold the nucleus in direct chop method.

Hyper Pulse Mode

In this mode the energy is delivered as that of burst mode, but more number of pulses will be delivered in each "ON" phase. For example if in burst mode it is 20 pulses per second, in hyper pulse mode it may be 120 pulses per second here we have the advantage of burst and linear modes. It is useful in emulsification of hard cataract by increasing the effectiveness of cutting by using only 50% of the energy. The heat generated also will be less. The surgeon can modify the number of pulses delivered per second depending on the hardness of the nucleus in a customized manner.

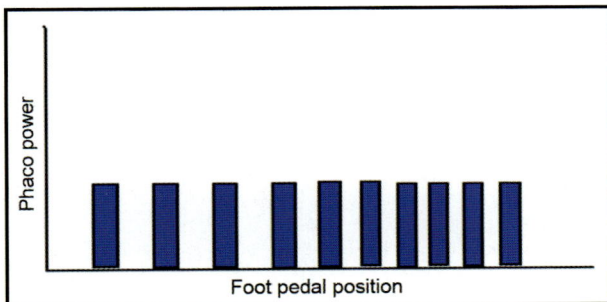

Fig. 19.6C: Burst mode—the preset energy is delivered even at the initial step of the footpedal

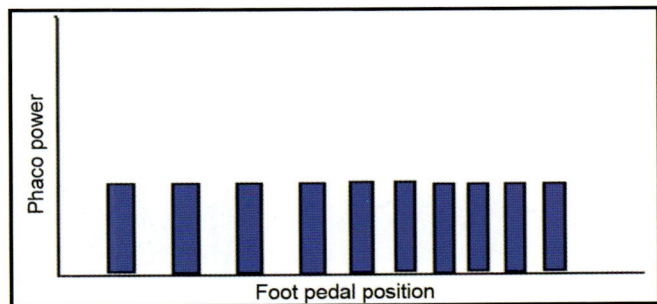

Fig. 19.6D: Hyper pulse mode

FLUIDICS IN AC

In Peristaltic Pump

Fluid currents in AC can be increased by increasing flow rate.

In Venturi Machine

Fluid currents in AC can be increased by increasing the vacuum.

By increasing the flow rate the effect is more prominent closer to the tip and is distributed in conical fashion.

By increasing the flow rate there is more attraction or fllowability and this acts as venturi pump in high flow rates.

The disadvantage of high flow rate is quick dragging of intraocular structures like iris and capsule and less reaction time for reflex.

Hence we recommend moderate flow rates which act mainly near the tip of phaco.

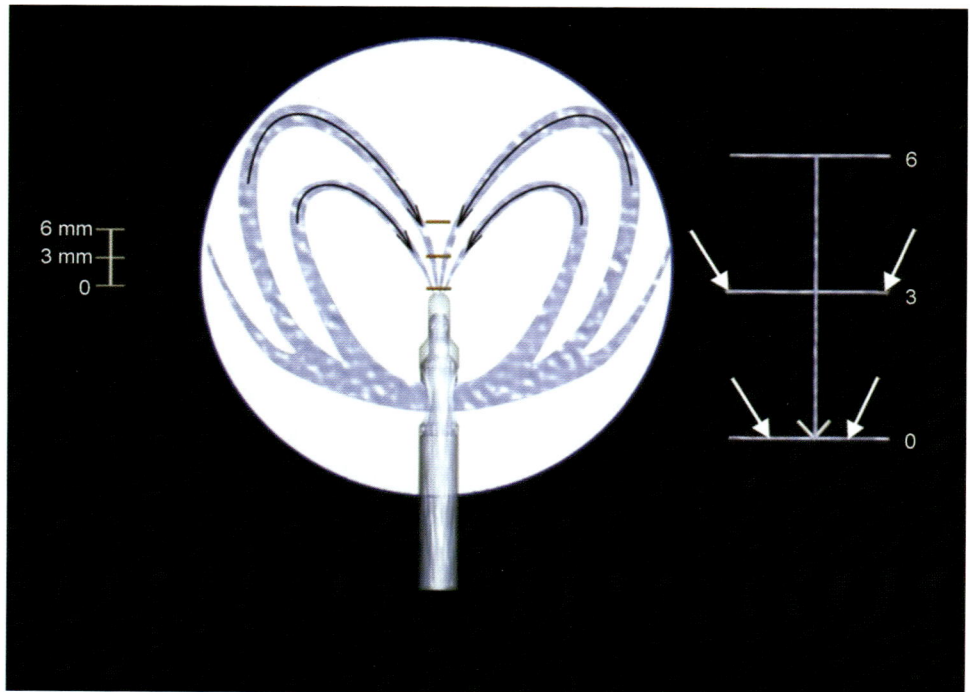

Fig. 19.7A: Close to the phaco tip at '0' the forces acting are more (4), at 3 mm point they are less (2) at 6 mm it is nil (0)

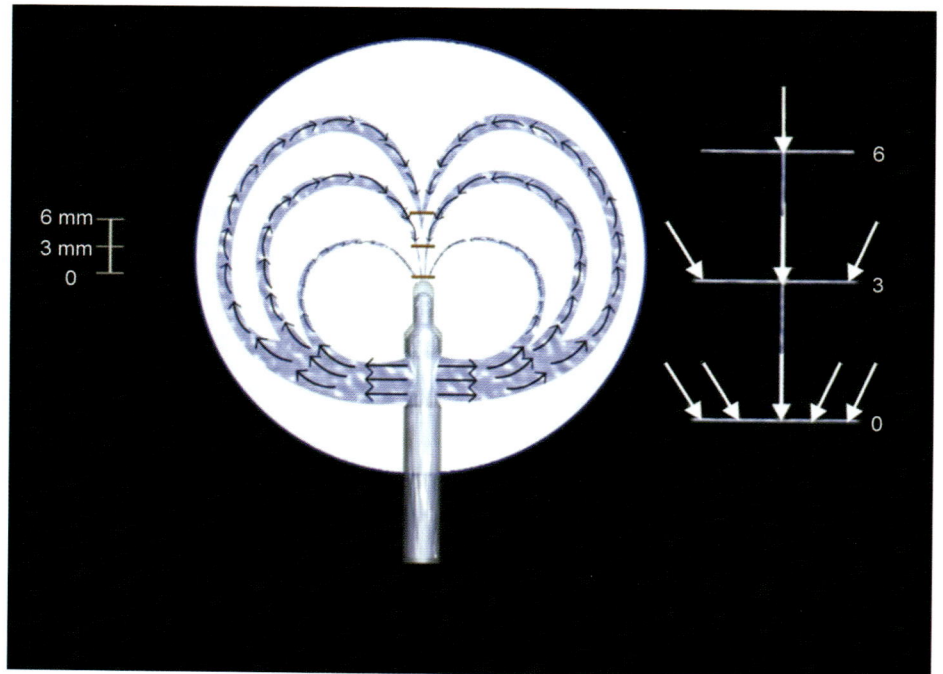

Fig. 19.7B: By increasing the AFR the fluidics (AC currents) are more, so by increasing the AFR, the peristaltic machine acts as venture machine. The fragments are attracted towards the tip

20

Phacotechnique

For Beginners

Select grade II and grade III nucleus. (Avoid too soft or too hard a nucleus)

Sclerocorneal incision: It is recommended to convert into SICS at any stage of surgery when the phaco procedure becomes uncomfortable.

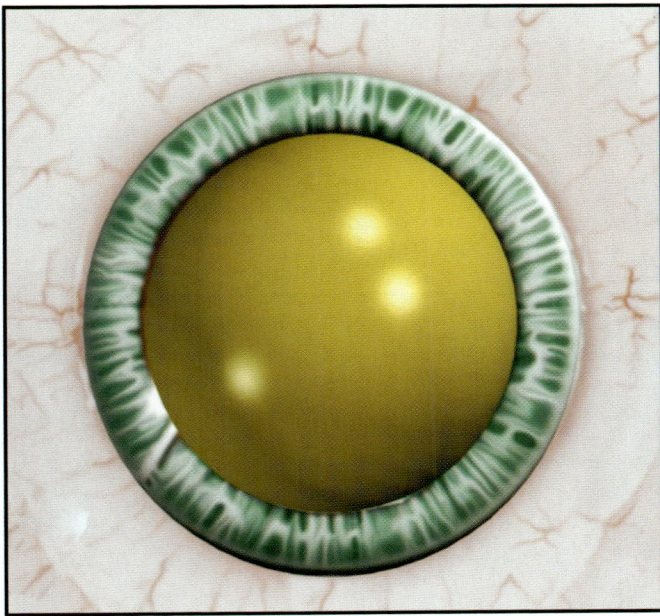

Fig. 20.1A: Sclerocorneal incision

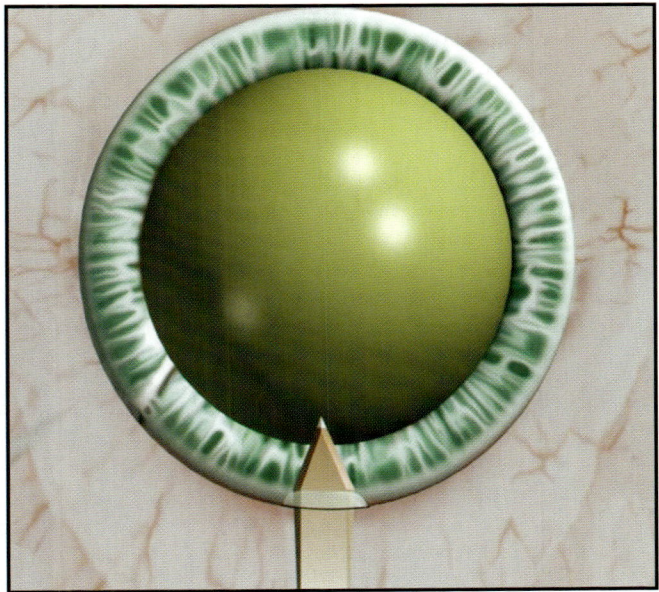

Fig. 20.1B: Clear corneal incision

Rhexis: Preferable to use dye (Trypan blue) as the blue not only stains and alters the fragility of the capsule but it also acts as a gauge for the surgeon to limit the , movement of the phaco tip.

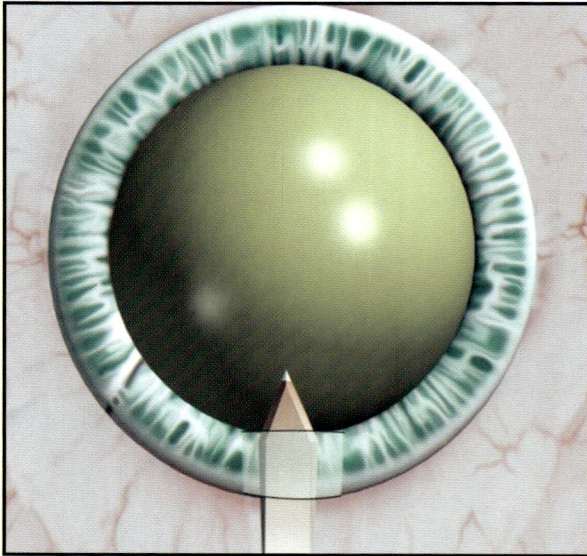

Fig. 20.1C: Near corneal incision

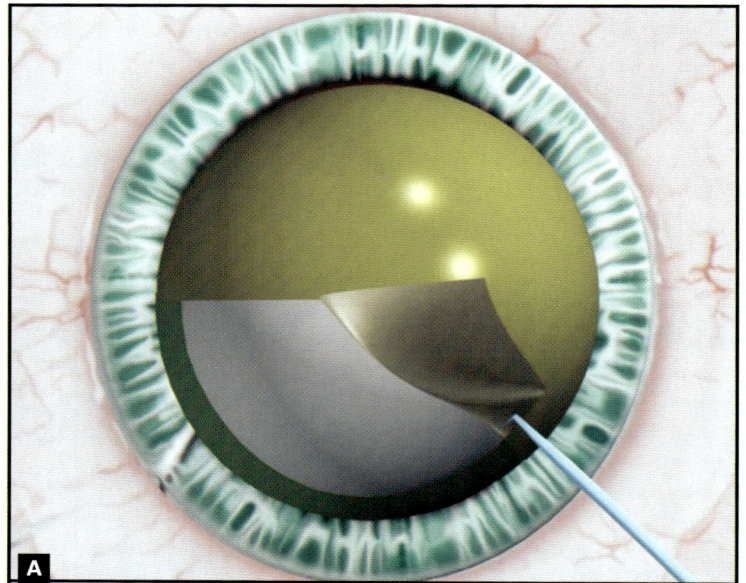

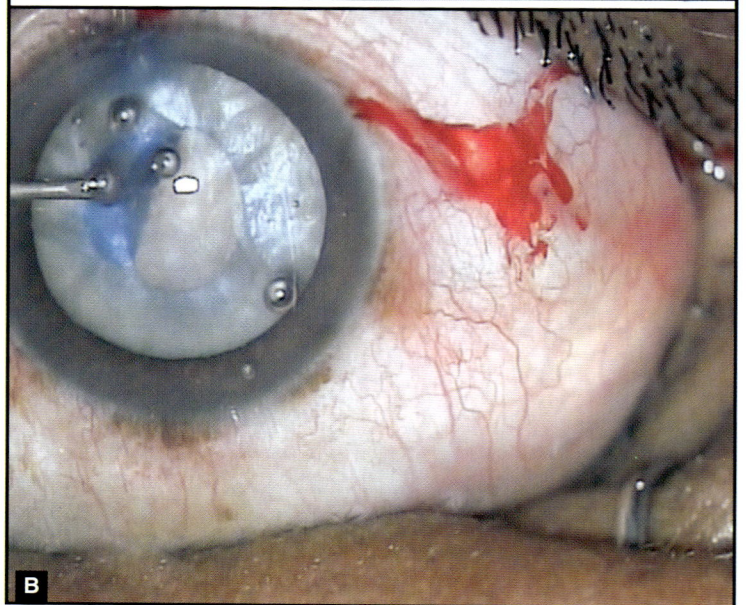

Figs 20.2A and B: CCC in the way

Hydroprocedure: Hydrodelineation is first done and hydrodissection is postponed till the nucleus is removed. The epinucleus and the cortex acts as a cushion during phaco.

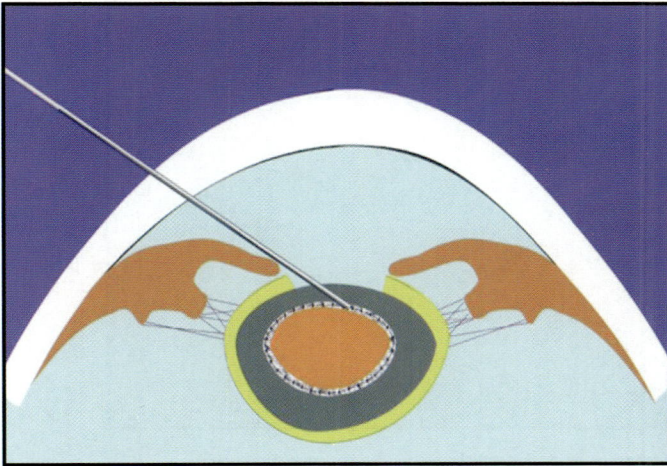

Fig. 20.3A: Hydrodelineation

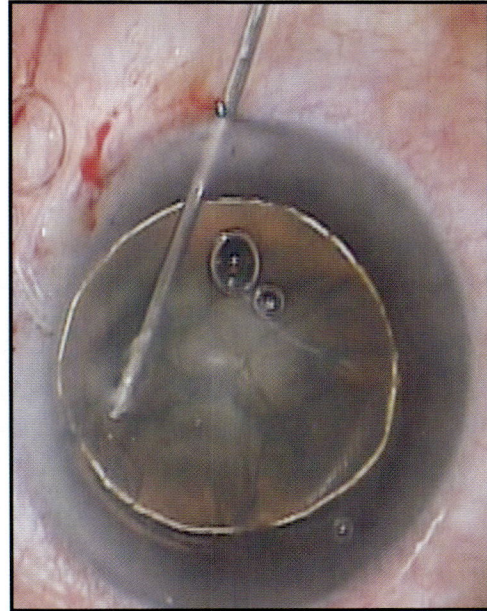

Fig. 20.3B: Golden ring appearance after hydrodelineation

Nucleus Management

Stop and Chop Technique

- The anterior chamber is filled with viscoelastic
- The lower half of the nucleus is grooved

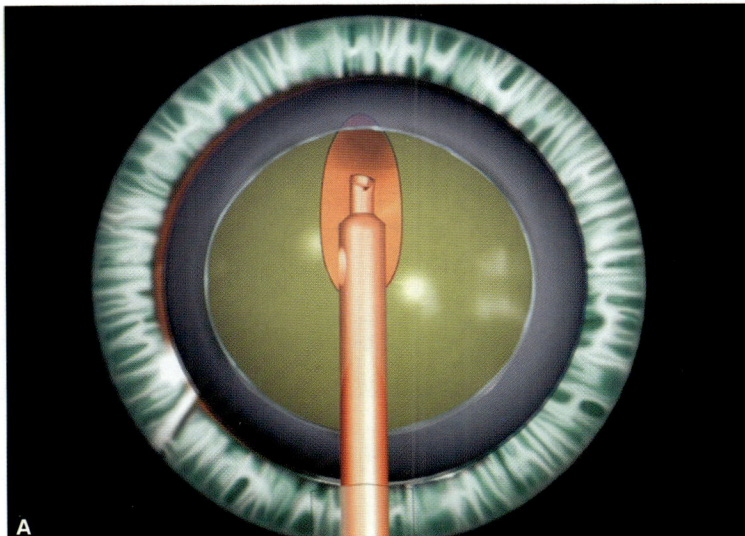

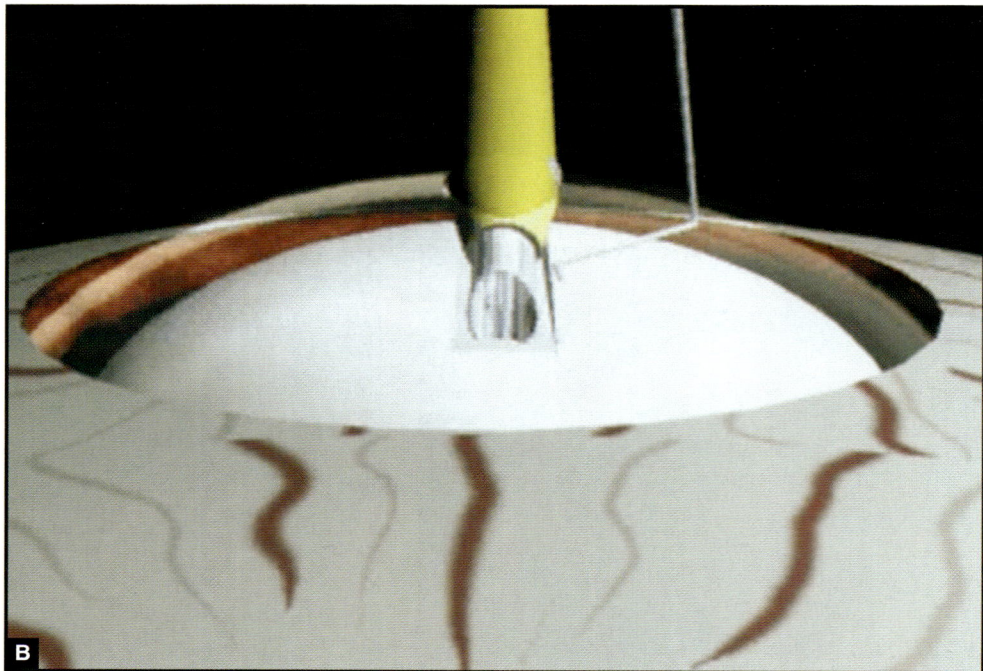

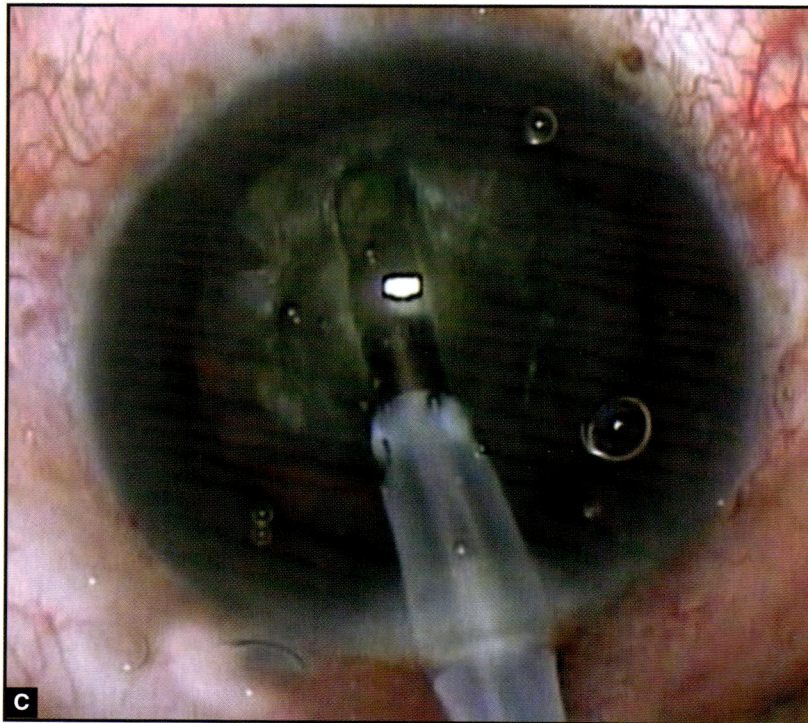

Figs 20.4A to C: Initial groove is made with phaco 1 in the lower half

• The nucleus is then rotated by 180° to complete the groove.

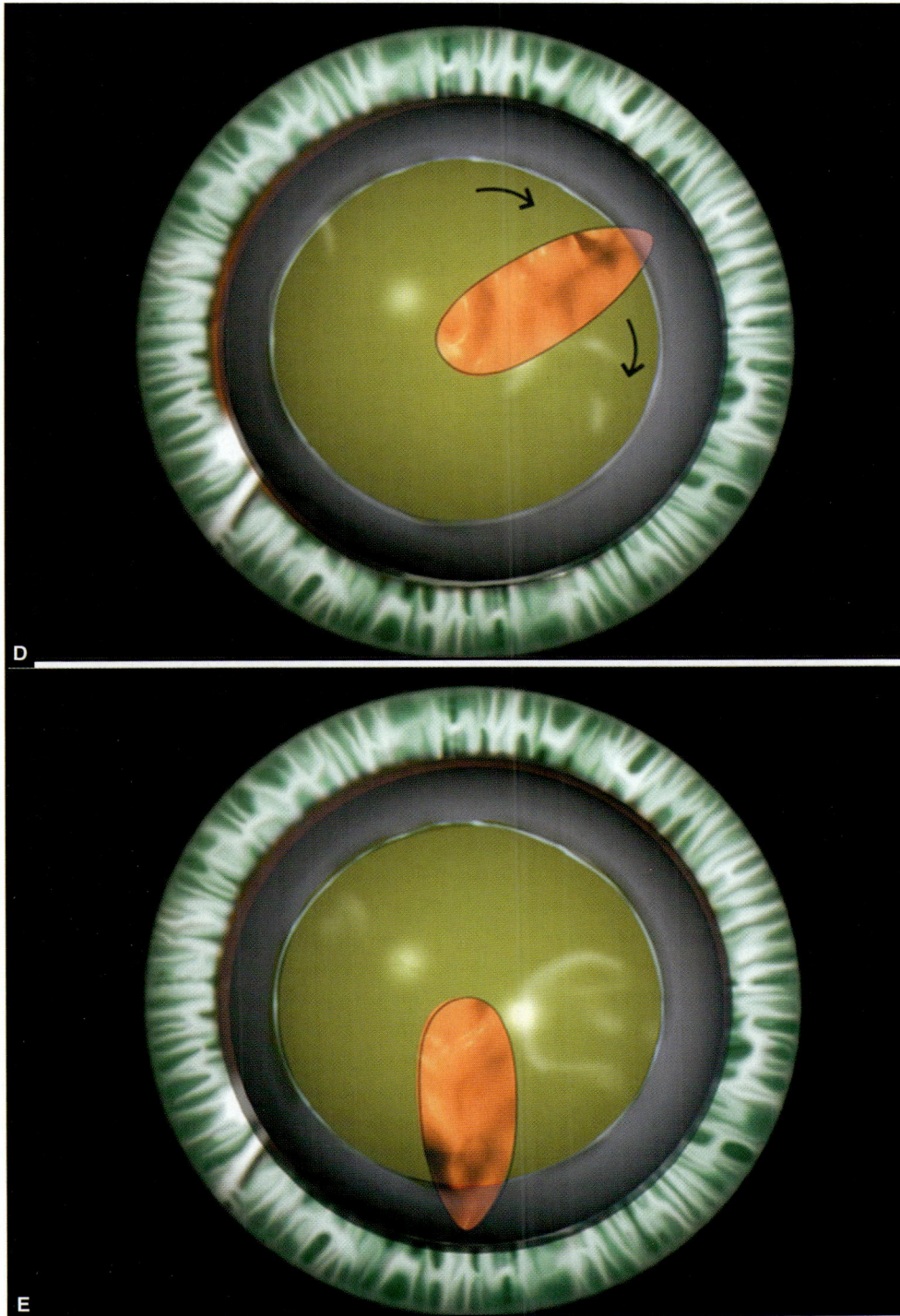

Figs 20.4D and E: 12 O' clock nucleus is rotated to 6 O' clock position

• Depth of the groove must be greater than 50%.

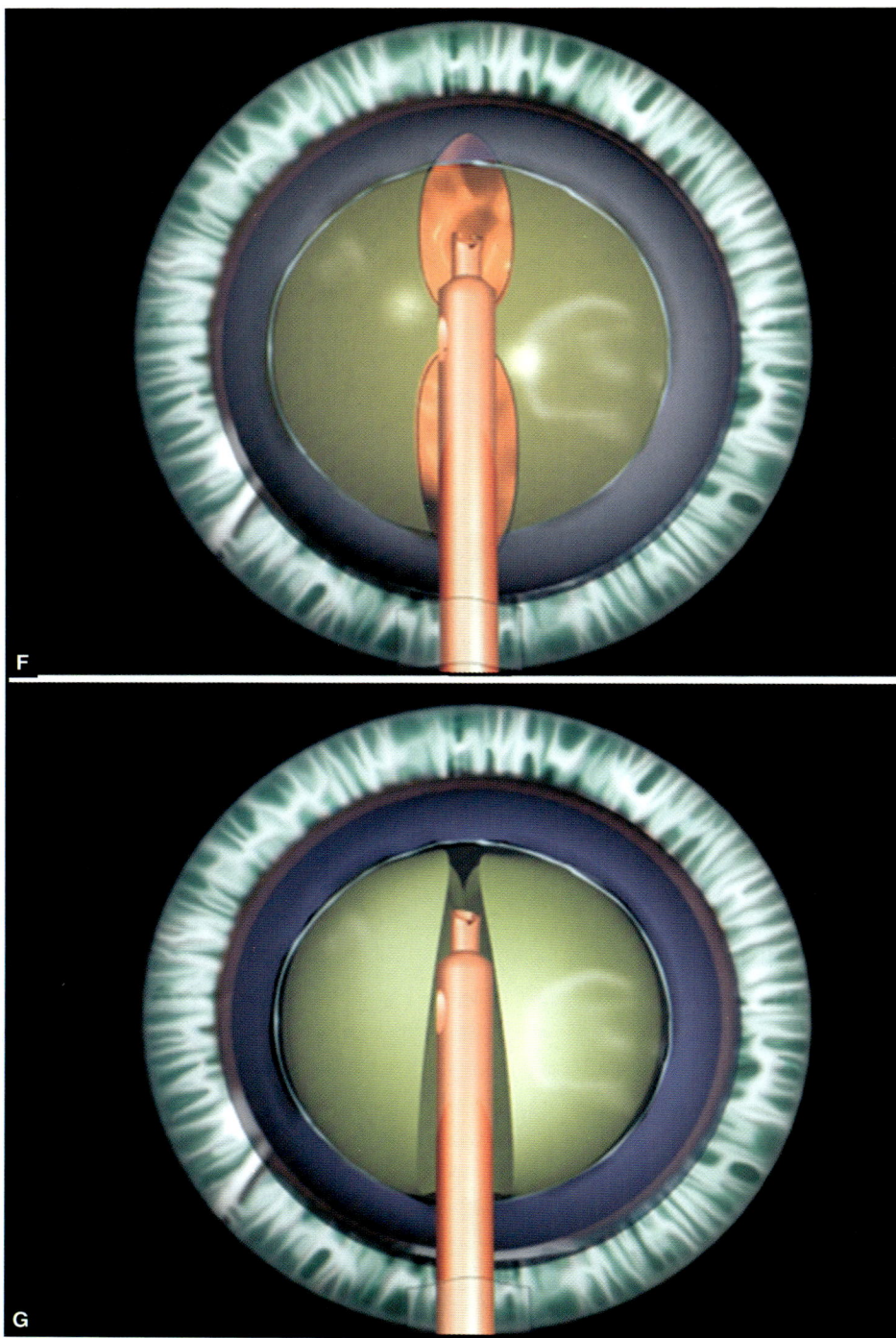

Figs 20.4F and G: Nuclear groove completed

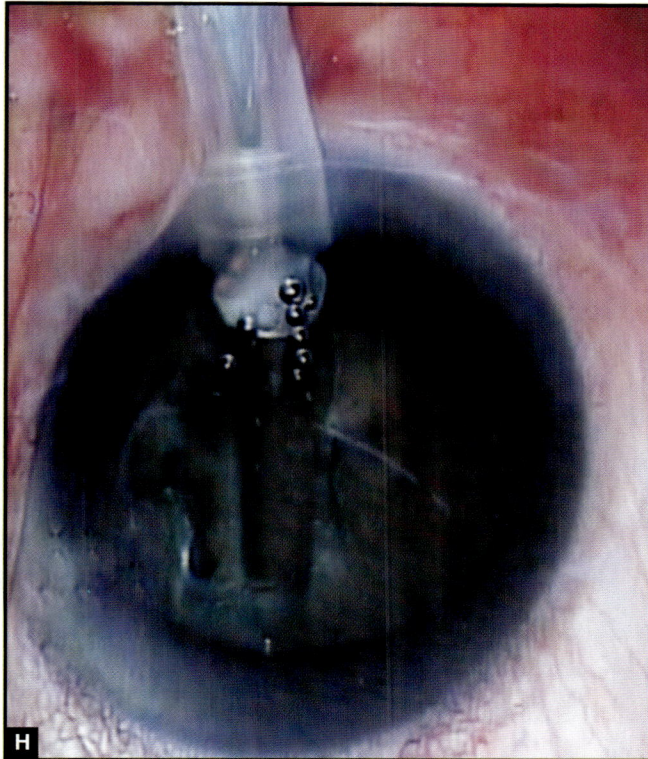

Fig. 20.4H: Trenching is done in other half to complete the groove and the groove is deepened

• Withdraw the phaco tip
• Take two choppers and divide the nucleus into two fragments.

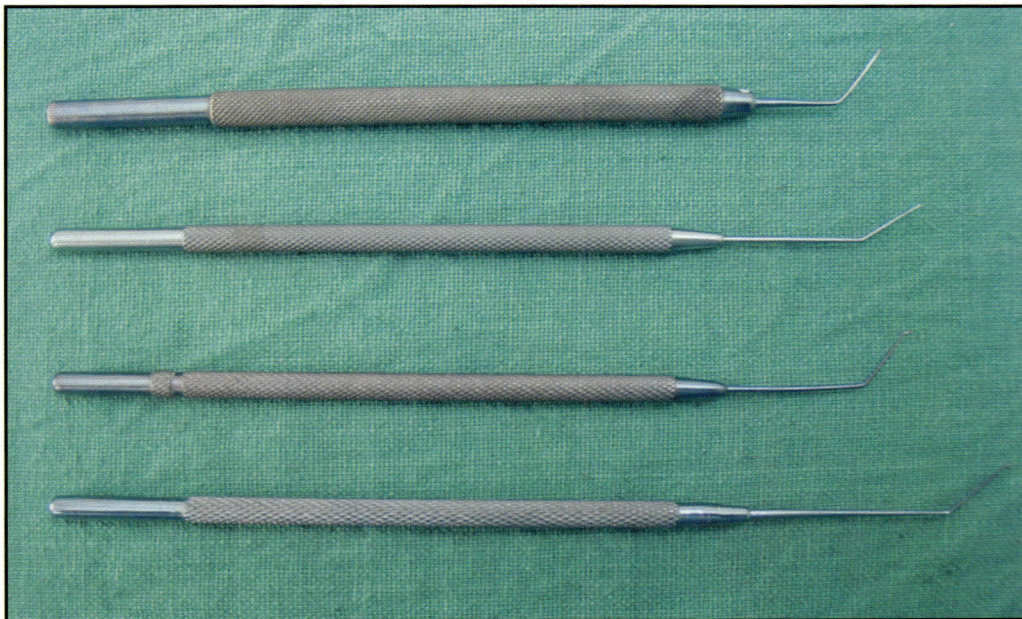

Fig. 20.4I: Choppers

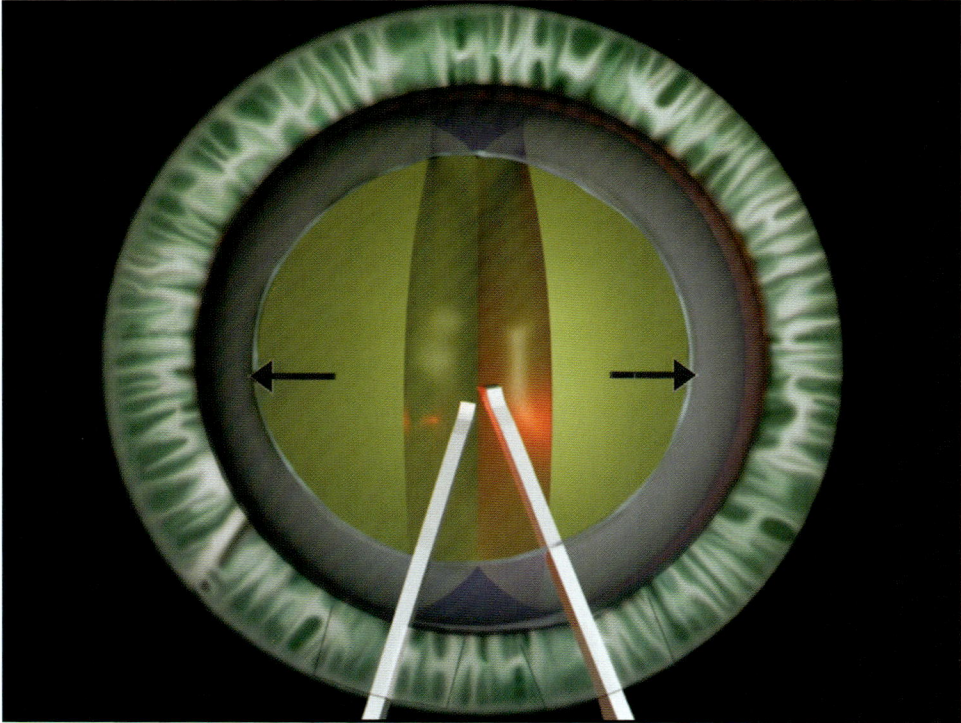

Fig. 20.4J: Nucleus being separated into two halves using choppers

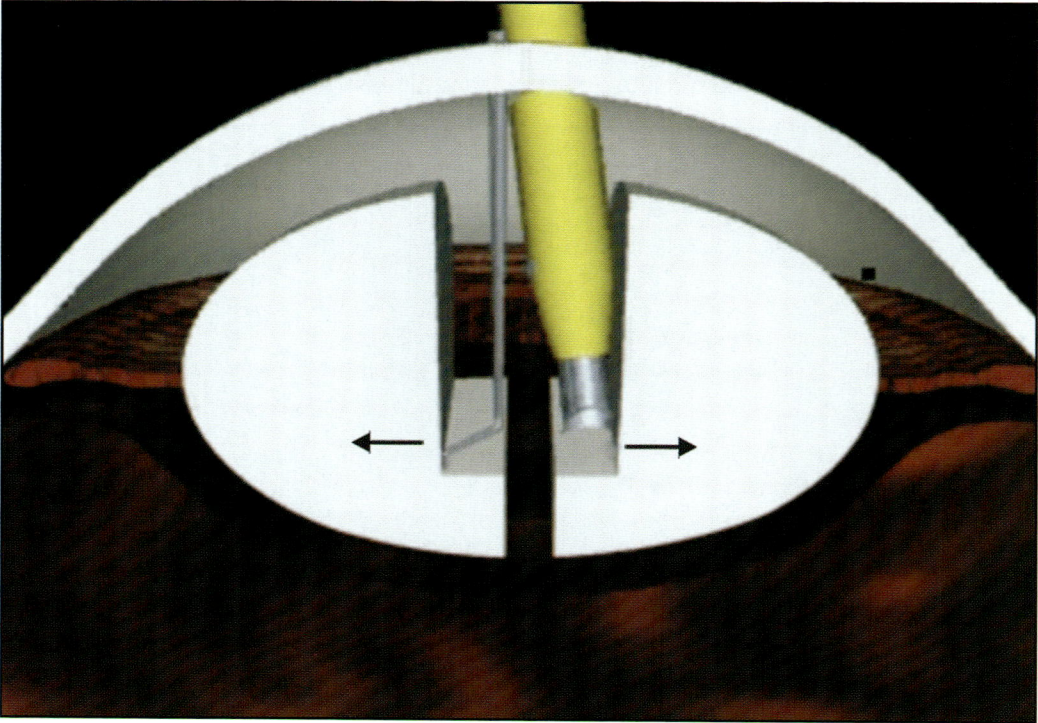

Fig. 20.4K: Nucleus can be divided into two halves with the use of the same phaco tip and chopper. Note that the two instruments should be at the bottom of the groove acting in opposite direction

- Care should be taken to see that all the small fibers are getting separated
- Inject viscoelastic into the anterior chamber
- Rotate the left fragment to 6 o' clock position and introduce the phaco with phaco II program (30% pulse, 25 cc, 300).

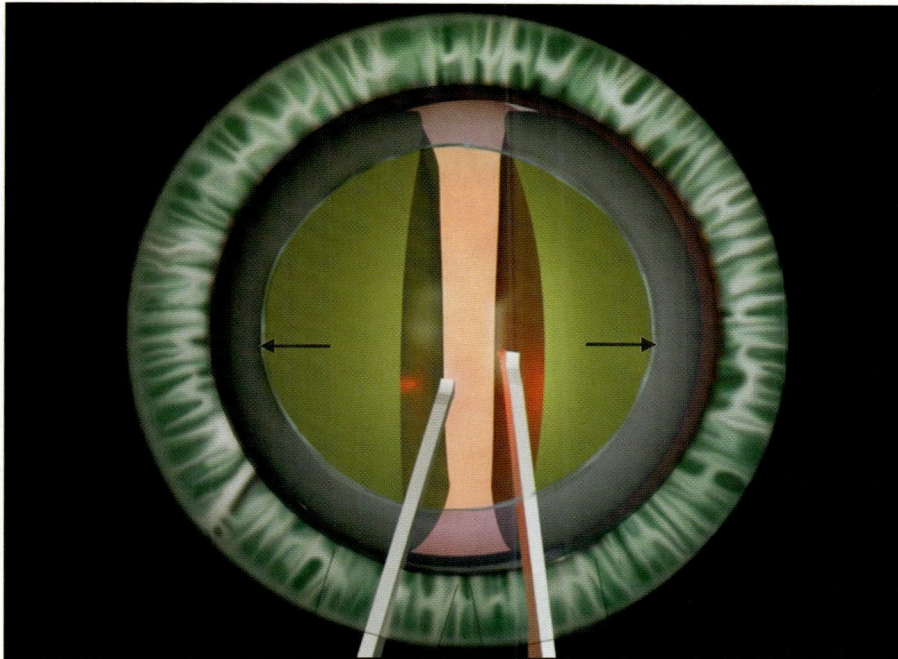

Fig. 20.4L: Two halves of nucleus are separated

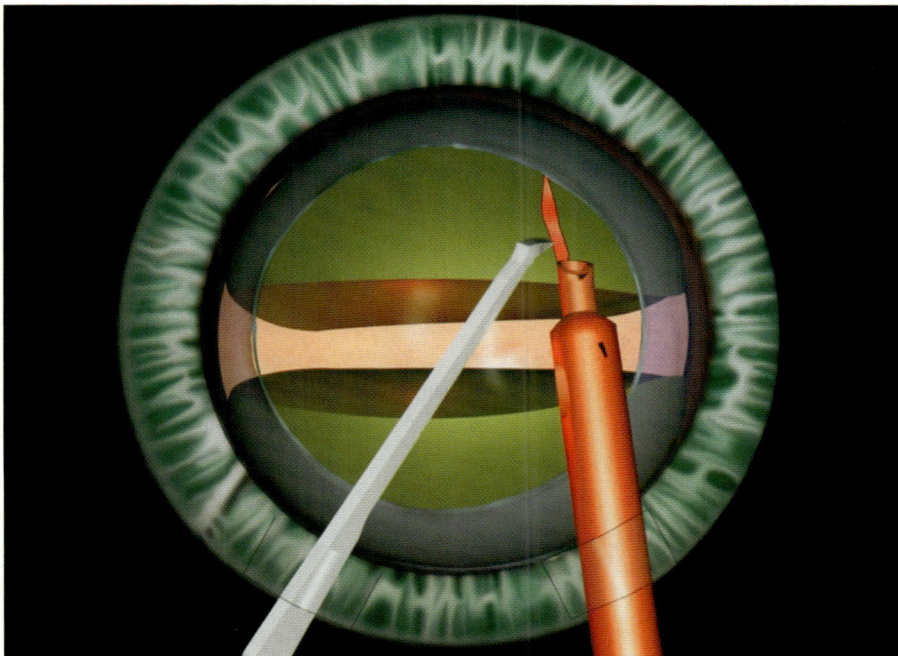

Fig. 20.4M: Two nuclear halves are in position so that one half is in the lower part

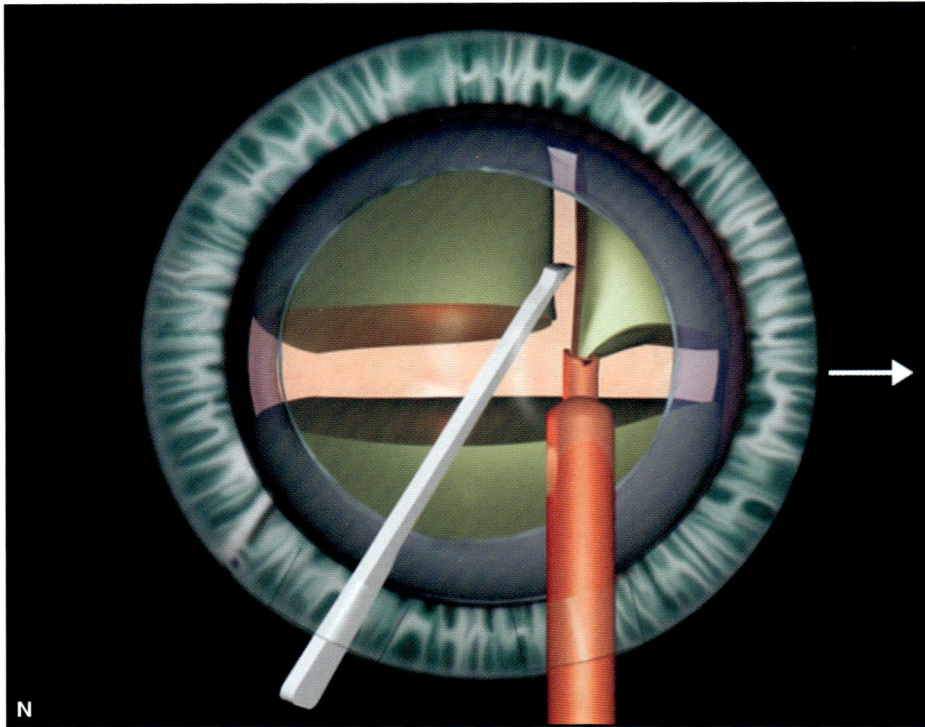

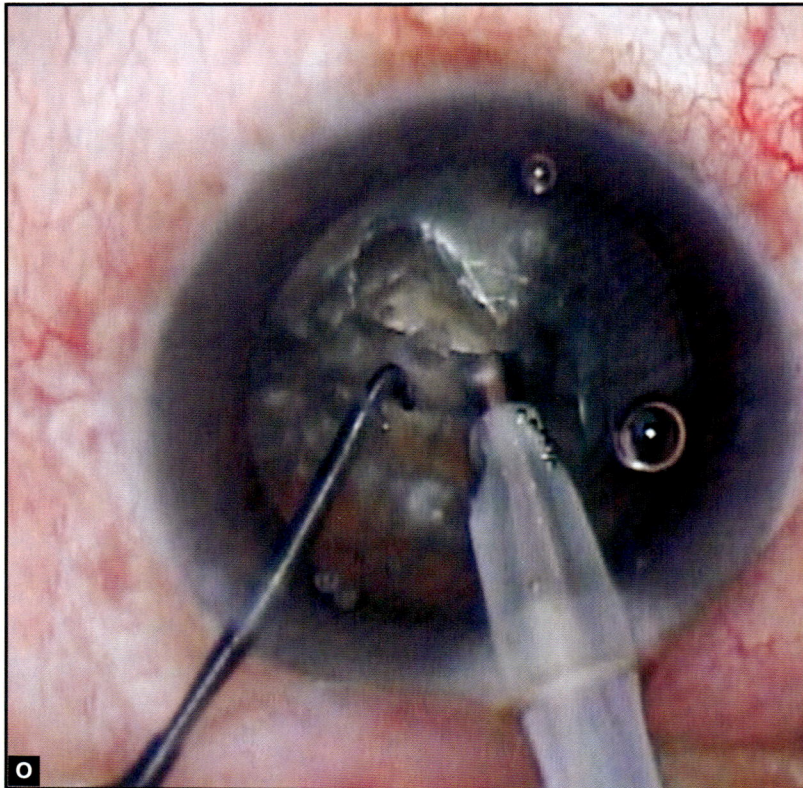

Figs 20.4N and O: Lower half is dealt using phaco II and chopper, nucleus is fragmented

- The main aim of phaco II is aspiration and holding of the fragments.
- With the help of the chopper, a number of fragments are made and these smaller fragments are aspirated using the pulse energy whenever necessary.

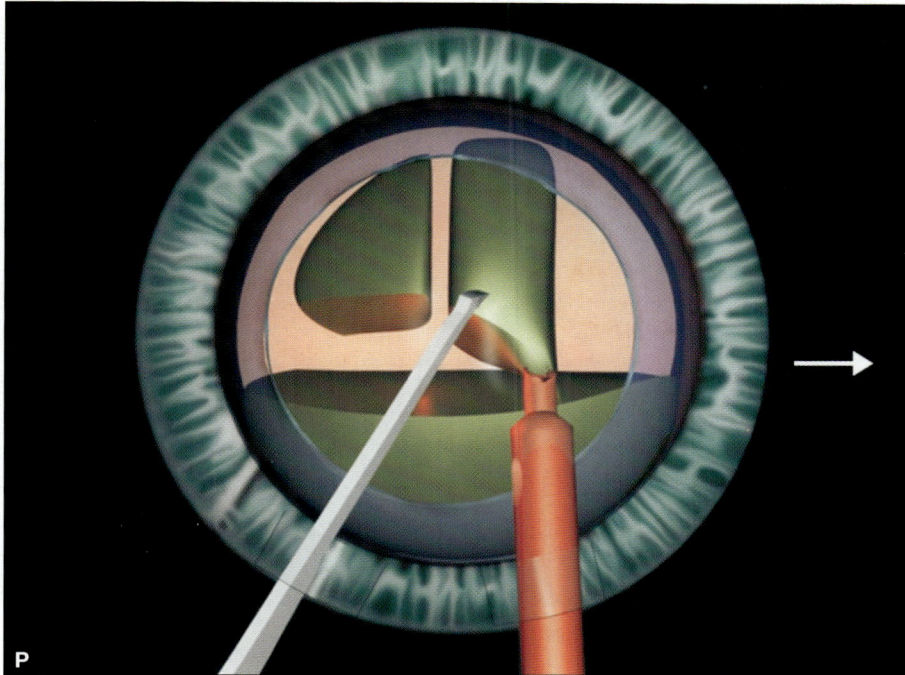

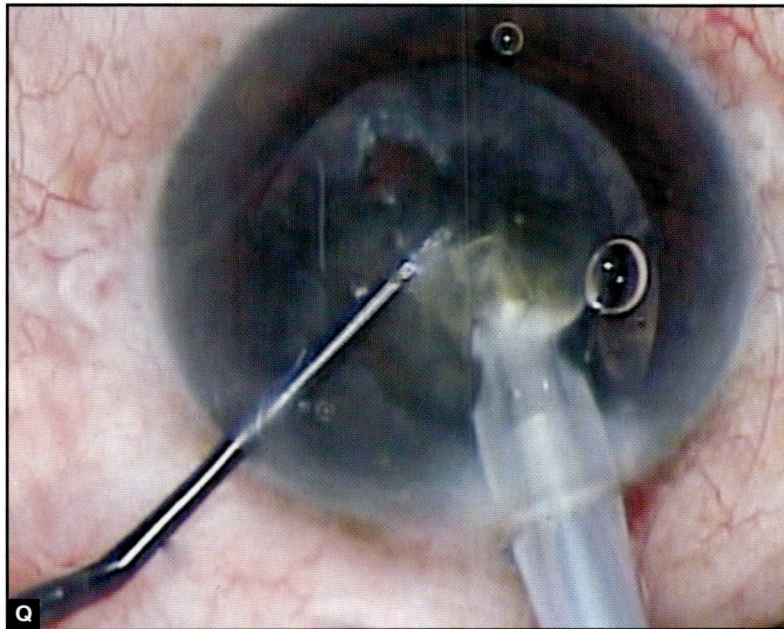

Fig. 20.4P and Q: Nucleus is made into as many fragments as possible and aspirated

- The other half of the nucleus is rotated to 6 O' clock position.

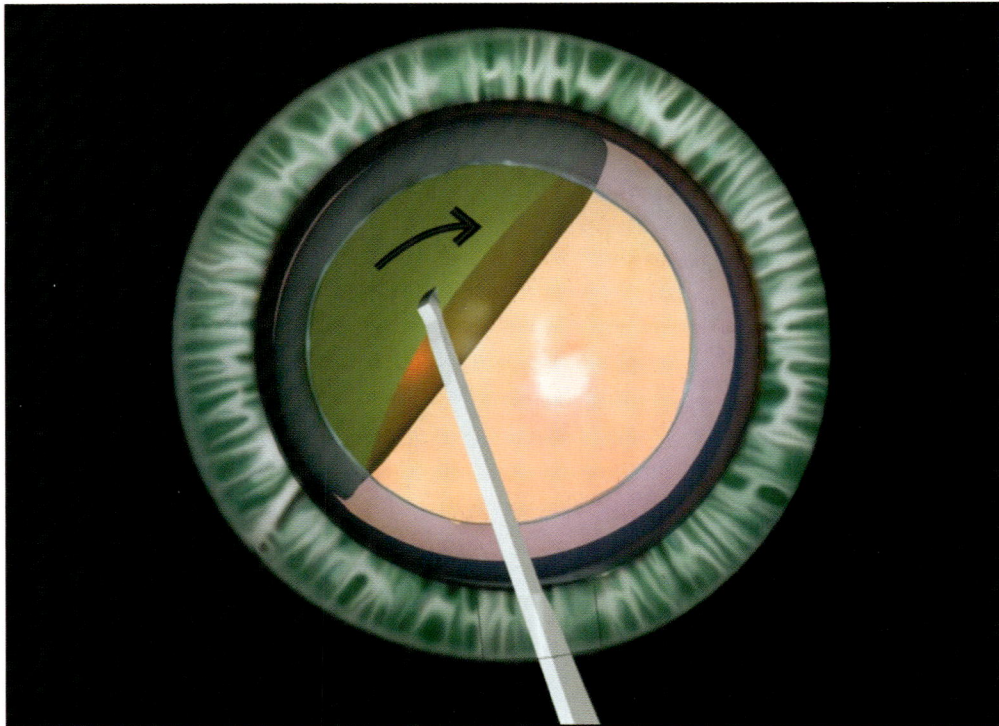

Fig. 20.4R: Rotation of the other half

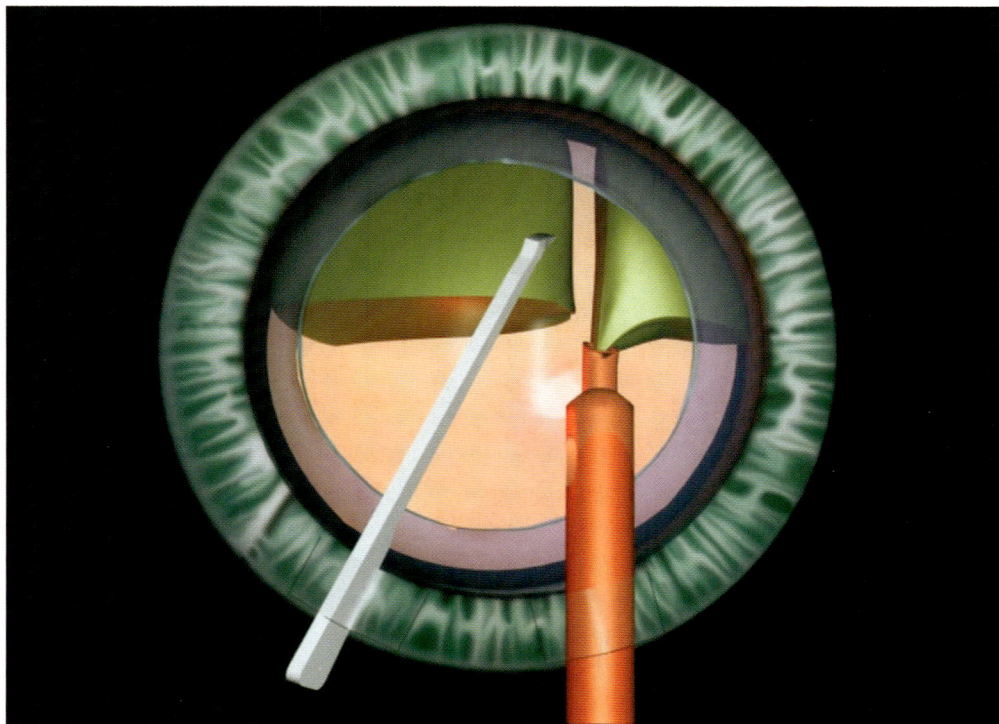

Fig. 20.4S: Fragmentation of the other half

• The same process of fragmentation and aspiration is repeated with the other half of the nucleus.

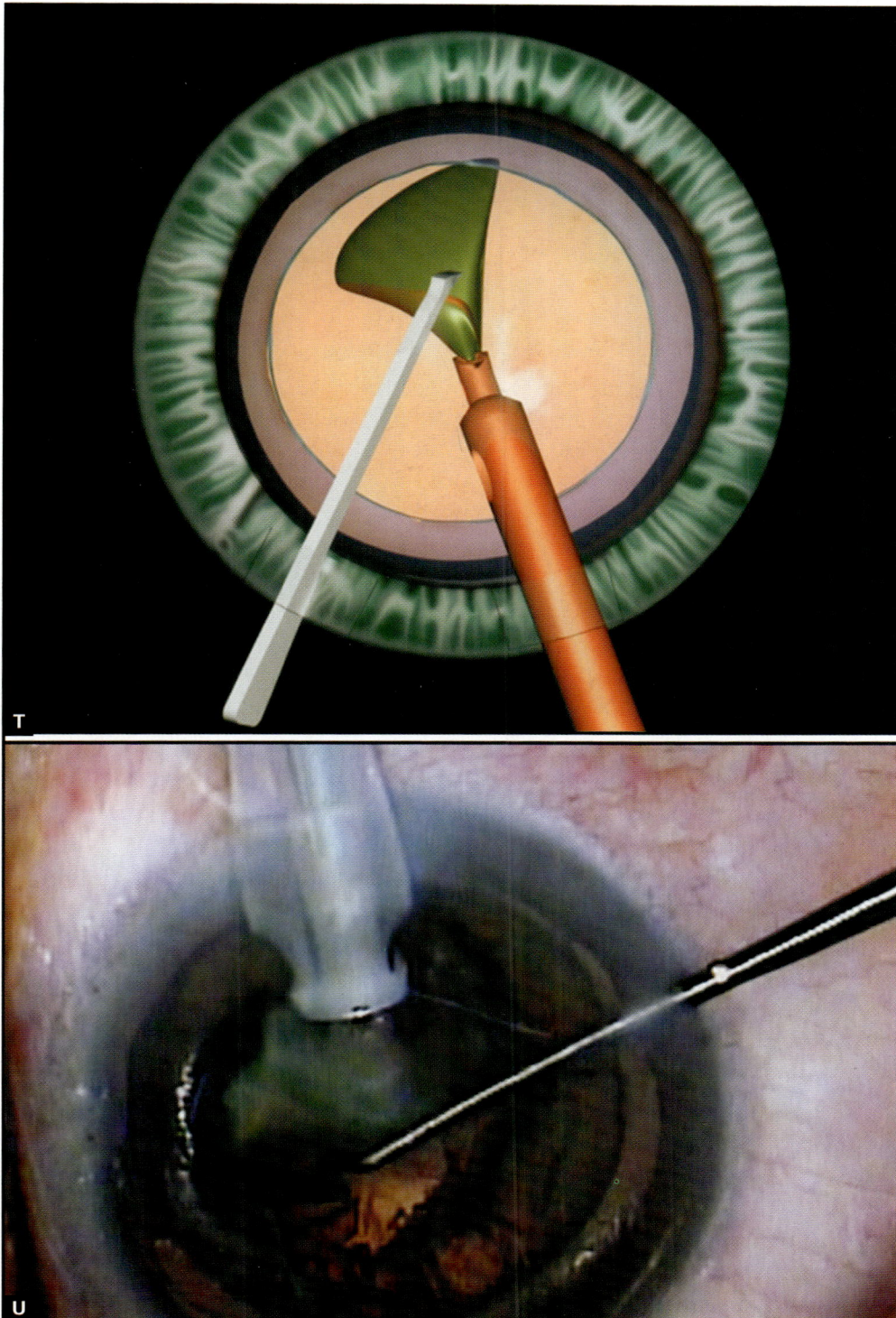

Figs 20.4T and U: Removal of the last fragment

- The remaining epinucleus is dislodged by injecting balanced salt solution beneath the capsule.
- The loose cortex and epinucleus will come to the center.

- In case of difficulty visco dissection is done
- Deepen the anterior chamber by injecting more visco
- The epinucleus is aspirated by phaco IV (Pulse 10%, 25 cc, 300)

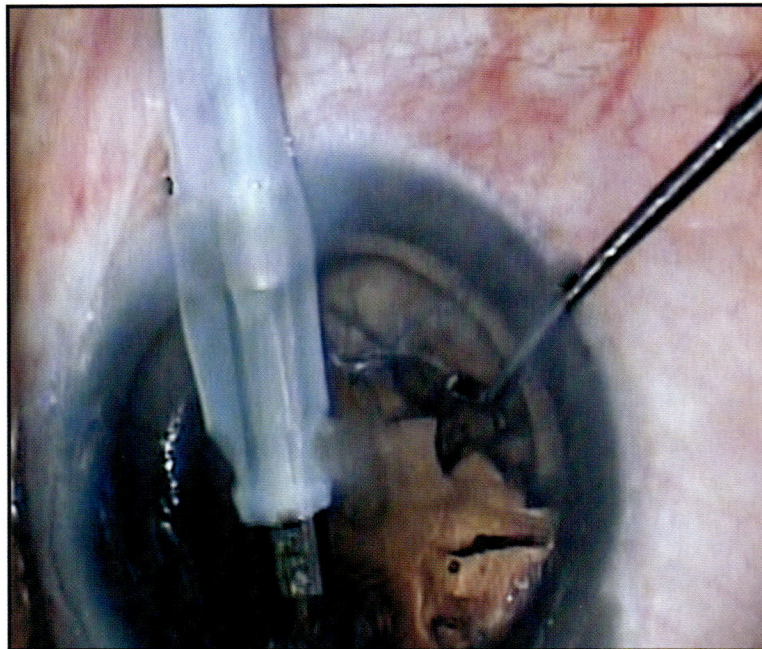

Fig. 20.4V: Removal of epinucleus using high vacuum (400 mm) and low phaco energy(10%)

- The remaining cortex is aspirated by bimanual irrigation and aspiration.

AUTHORS CHOICE OF PHACO PROCEDURE

Direct Chop Technique

Clear Corneal Incision: Site: Depends on the steeper meridian
- If K1 (horizontal) is more, temporal incision is taken
- If K2 (vertical) is more, 12 O' clock incision is taken.

Side Entry: Two side entries are made at 10 O' clock and 2 O' clock using 20 gauge MVR blade after overfilling the anterior chamber with viscoelastic substances.

Capsulorhexis

- This is achieved using 26 gauge needle mounted on a visco syringe
- The size of the rhexis is 5.5 mm as the size of the IOL is 6 mm.

Hydroprocedure

- Hydrodissection and hydrodelineation are done
- Check for the free movement of the nucleus
- In case of nuclear cataract do not do forceful rotation of the nucleus as it might cause zonular rupture or posterior capsular rent.

Nucleus management

Phacoemulsification (AMO sovereign) Table 20.1 Phaco Parameter

Mode	Power	AFR	Vacuum
Phaco I	70%	25 cc	25 mm Hg
Phaco II	30%	25 cc	300 mm Hg
Phaco III	Burst mode	25 cc	300 mm Hg
Phaco IV	10%	25 cc	300 mm Hg
I and A	— —	25 cc	400 mm Hg
Capsule polishing	— —	25 cc	20 mm Hg

Sculpting and Trenching

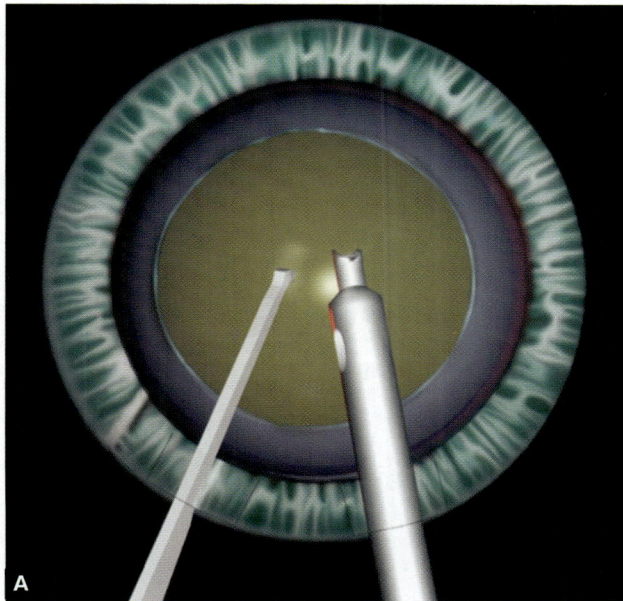

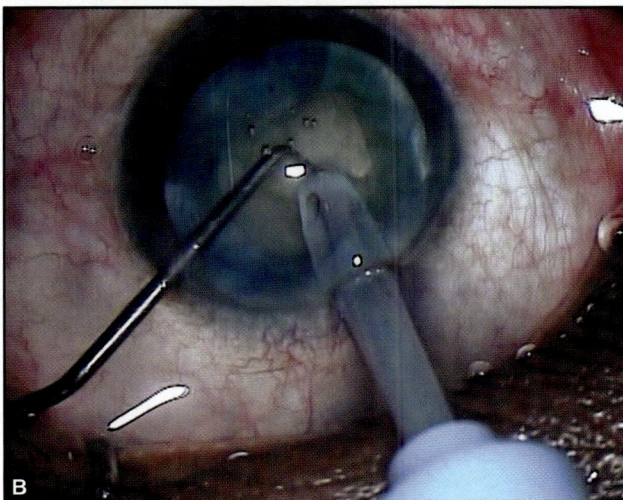

Figs 20.5A and B: Phaco probe is burried into the center of nucleus with burst mode

- If the cataract is soft direct trenching in two or three strokes is enough
- Next divide the nucleus into two or three fragments and keep the phaco in phaco II position and aspirate the fragments.

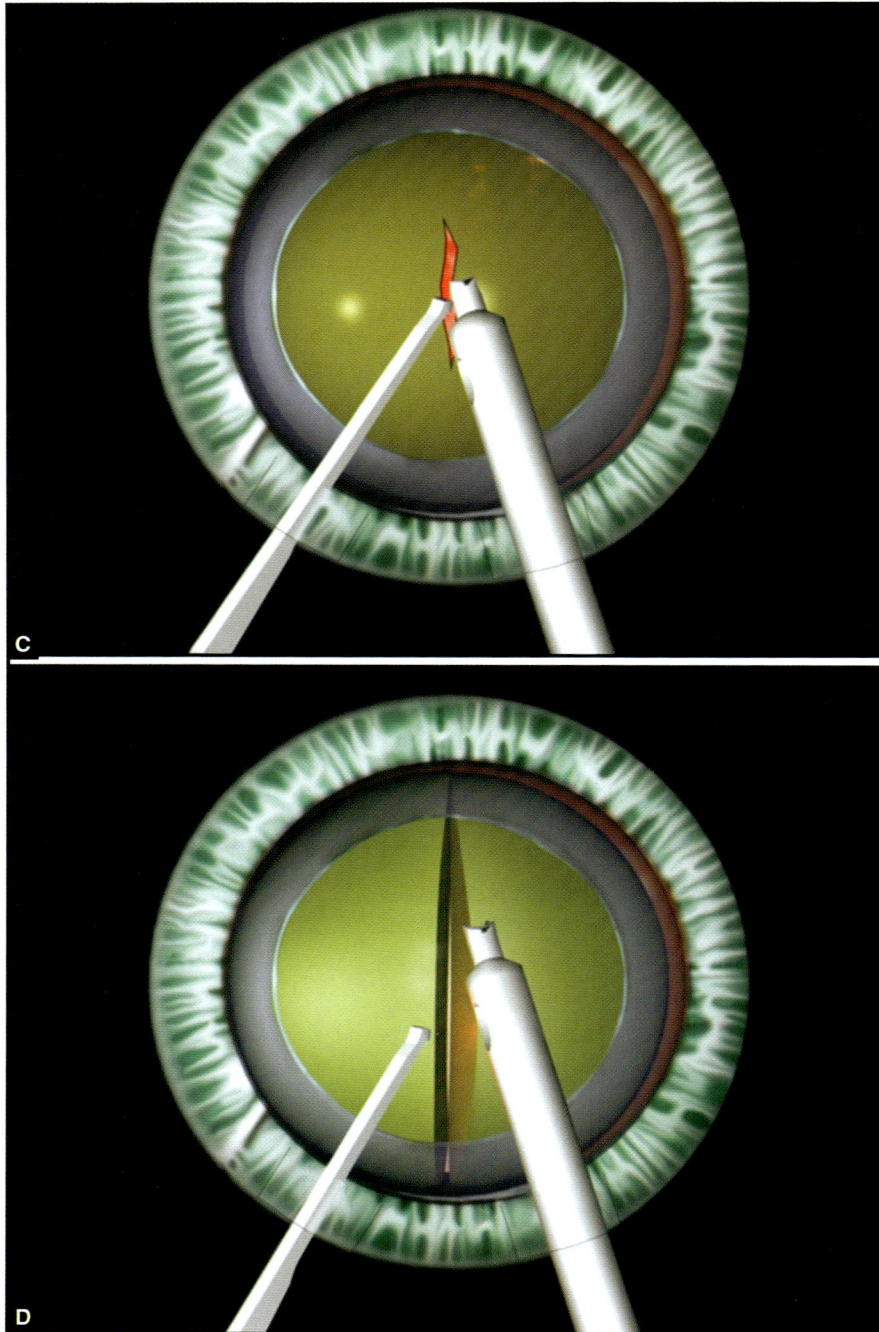

Figs 20.5C and D: Choppers moved from 6 O' clock to 12 O' clock with minimal lateral pressure and the nucleus is cracked

- If necessary, make them smaller using the chopper
- If the cataract is hard sculpting and trenching is done to create central space

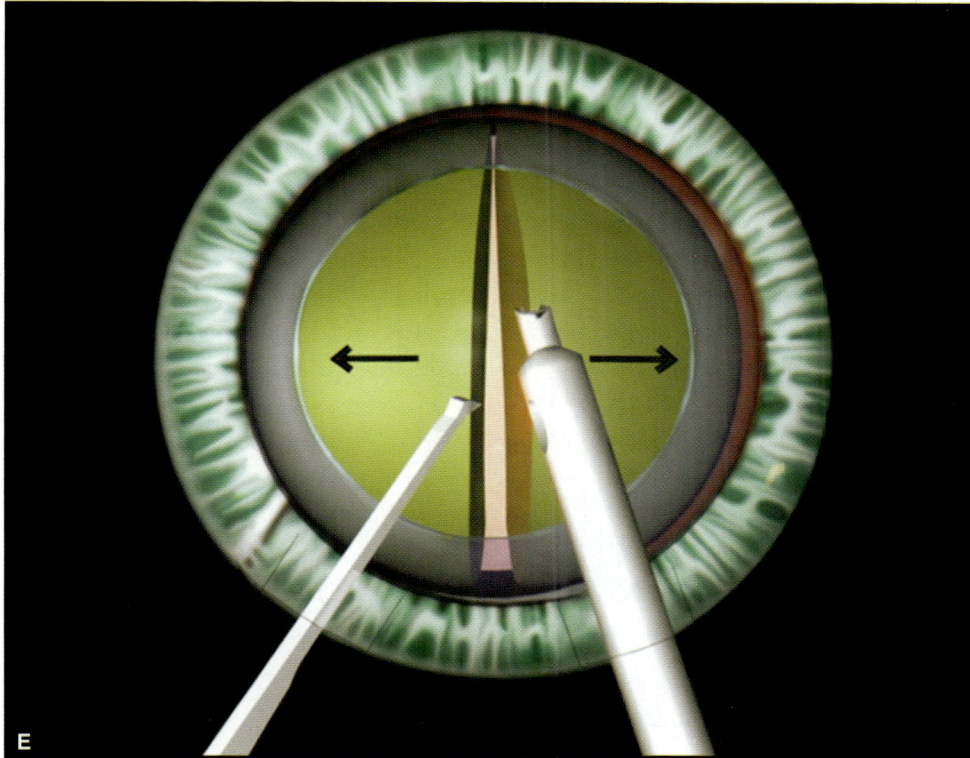

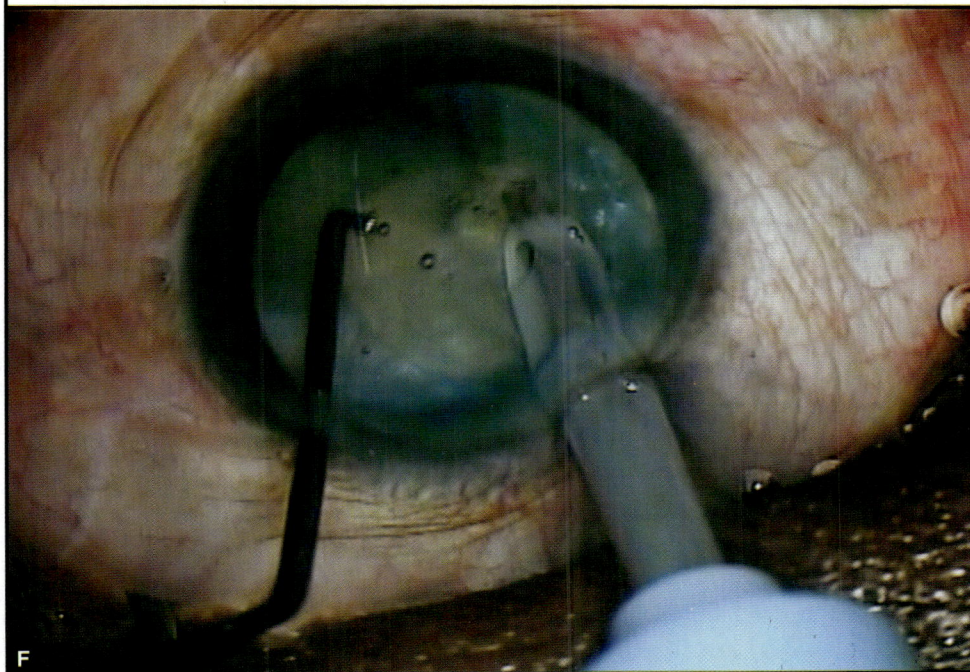

Figs 20.5E and F: Chopper is burried into the groove for easy separation

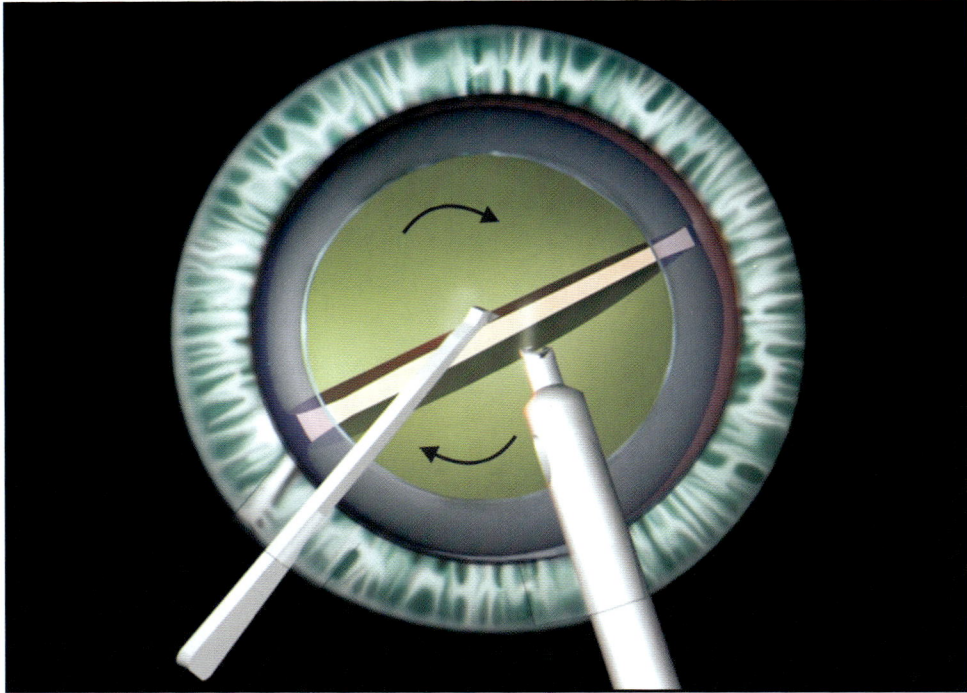

Fig. 20.5G: Fragments are rotated to position one half of nucleus in the lower part

- Then turn to burst mode and crack the nucleus with single pulse into pieces
- Repeat the same until we get a number of pieces
- Emulsify the same in the bag

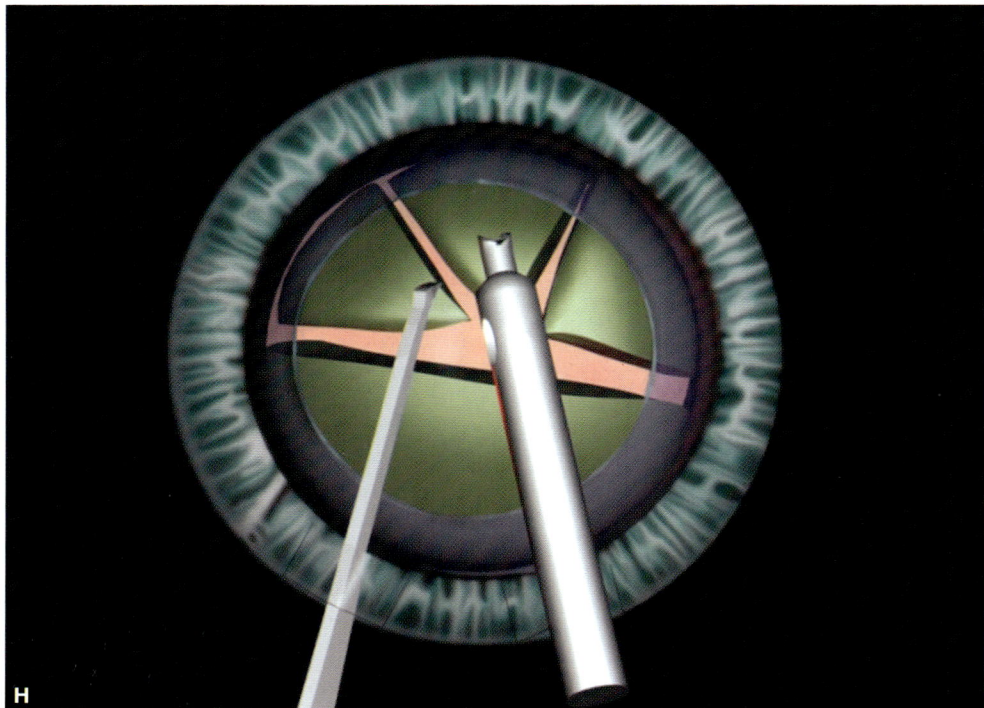

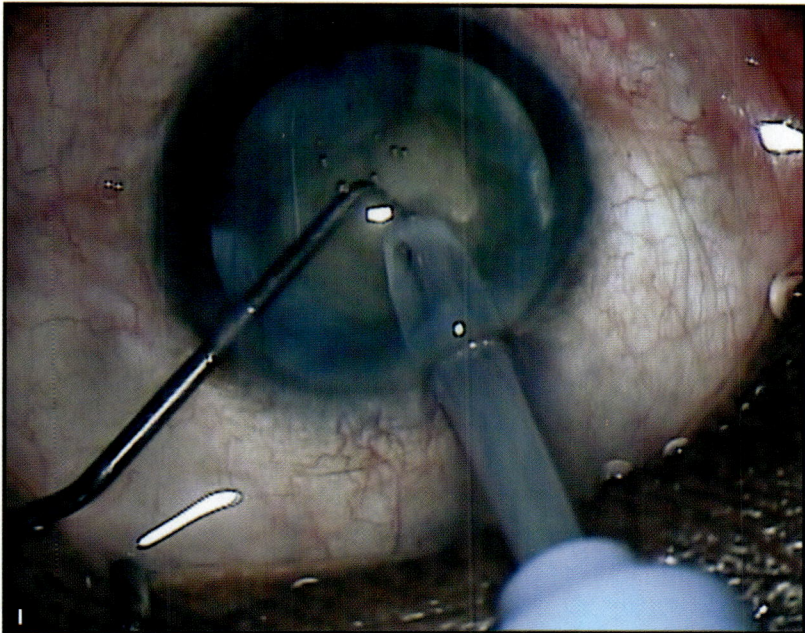

Figs 20.5H and I: Each half is made into multiple fragments

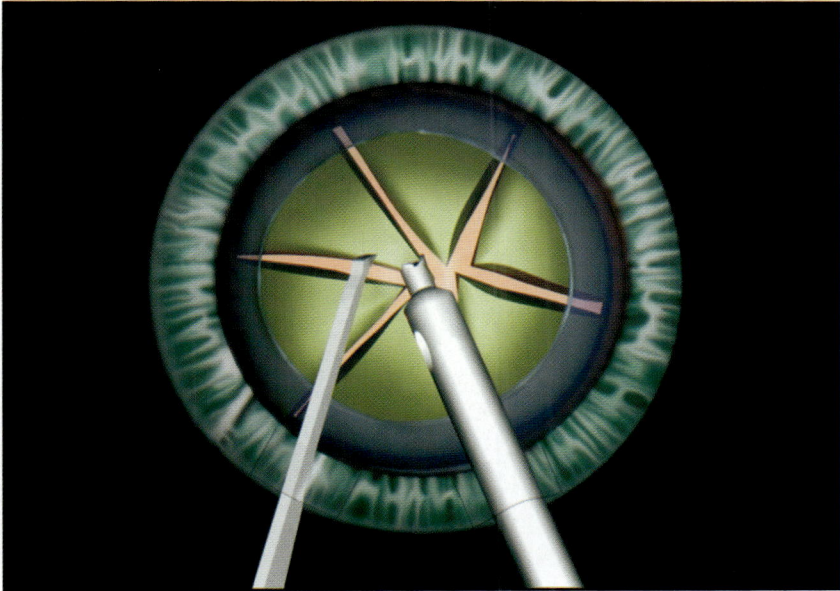

Figs 20.5J: Multiple fragments are made like pie of a pizza

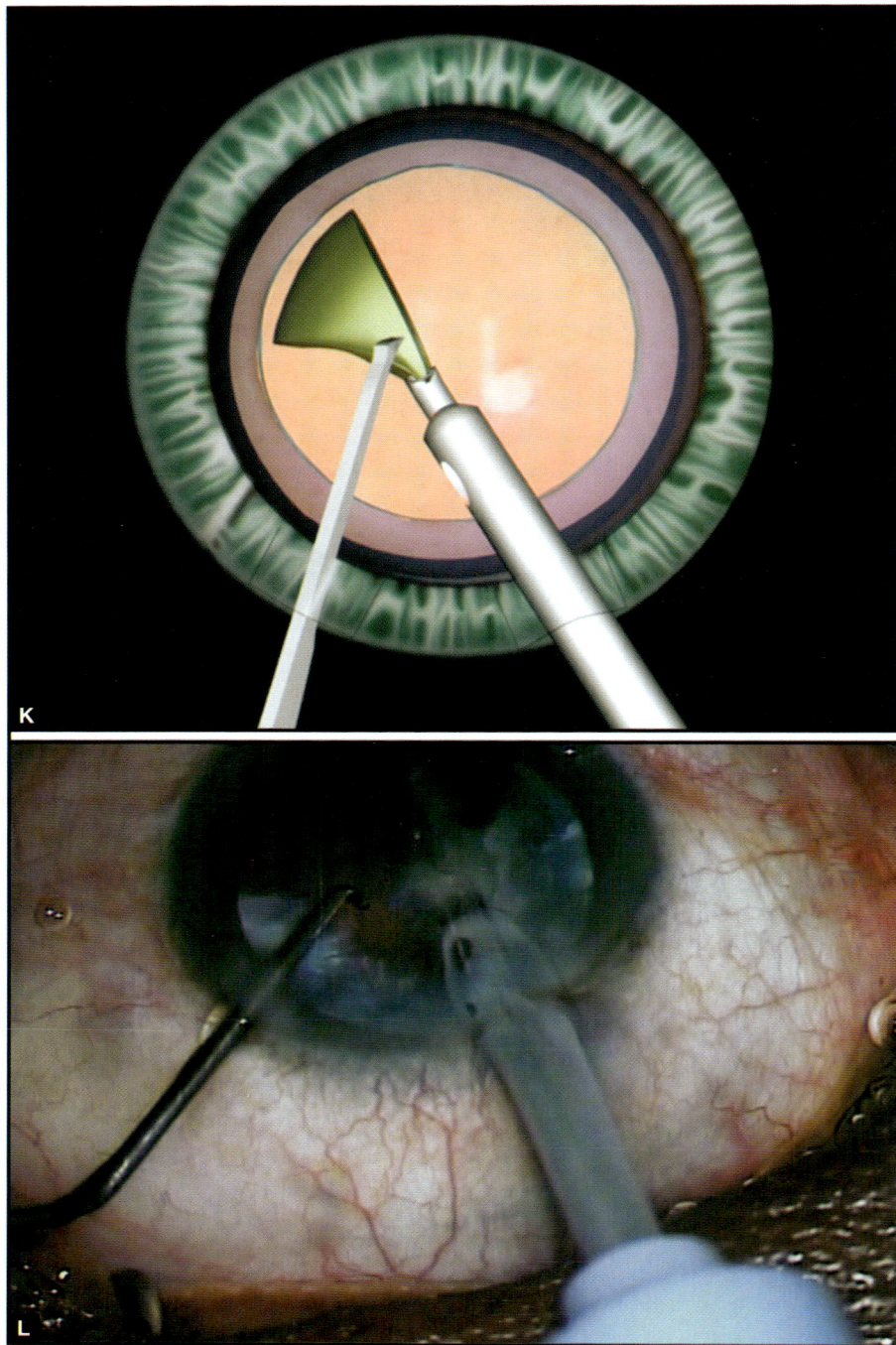

Figs 20.5K and L: Removal of last fragment with low aspiration 2 low vacuum

- Irrigation and aspiration is done using bimanual cannula

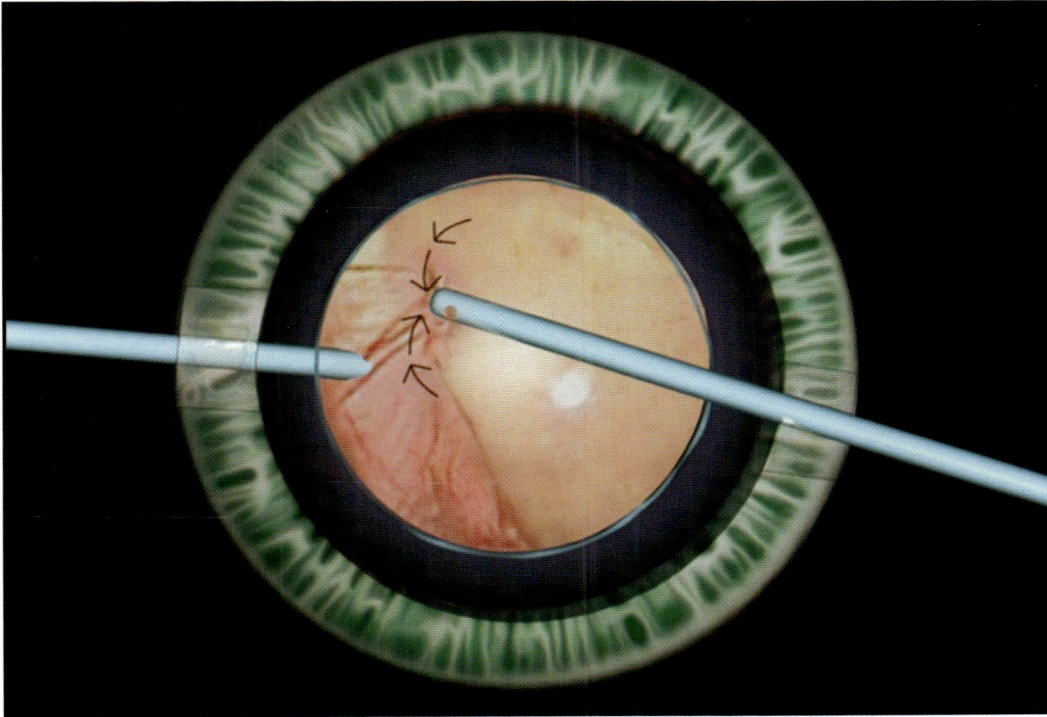

Fig. 20.6A: Removal of one half of cortex using bimanual I and A

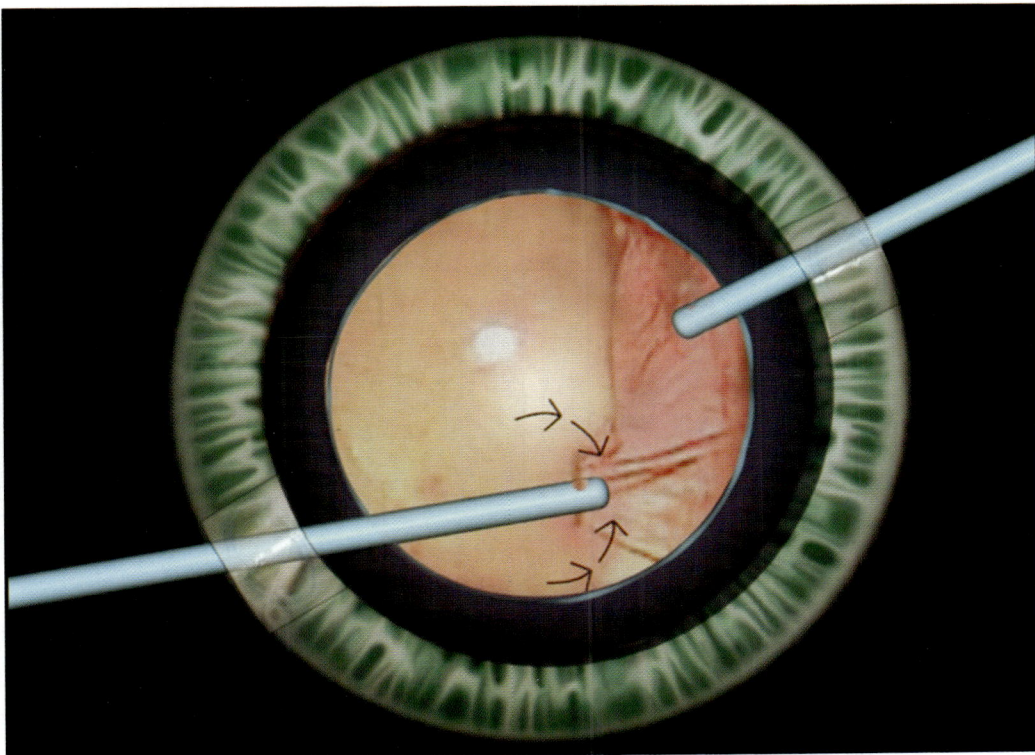

Fig. 20.6B: Removal of other half of cortex

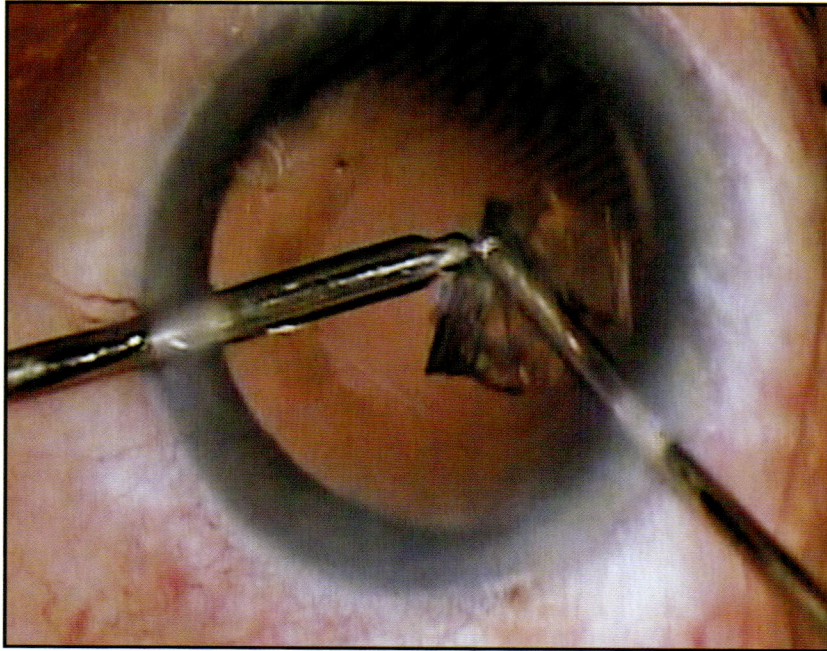

Fig. 20.6C: Cortical removal with bimanual I and A

IOL placement

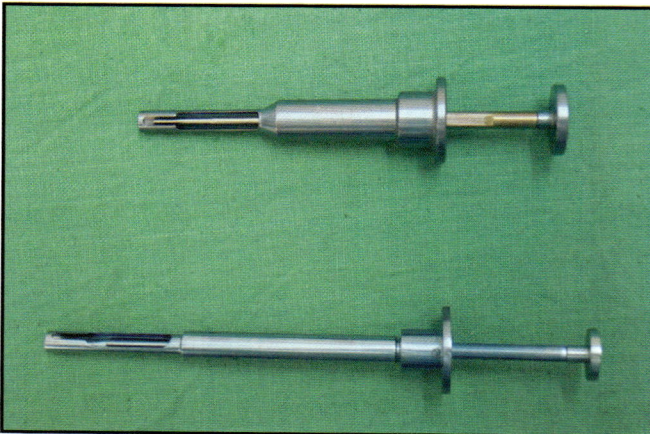

Fig. 20.7A: Injectors for foldable IOLs

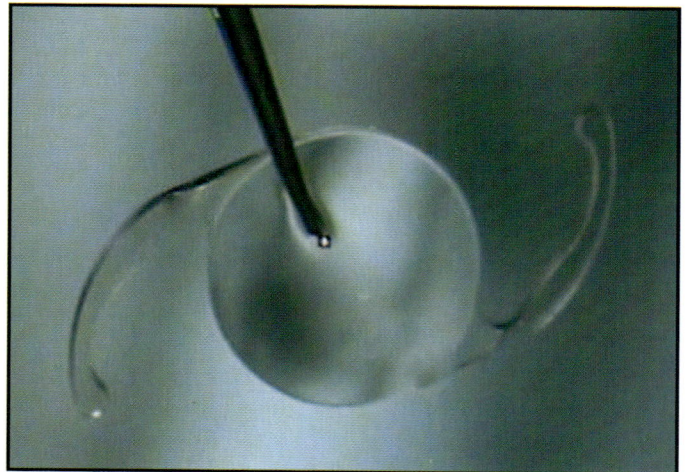

Fig. 20.7B: Foldable IOL, Acrysof

Foldable IOL is placed in the bag

- The IOL is placed in the bag taking care that the leading loop goes into the bag and the IOL is dialed turning the haptic with the help of a Y hook

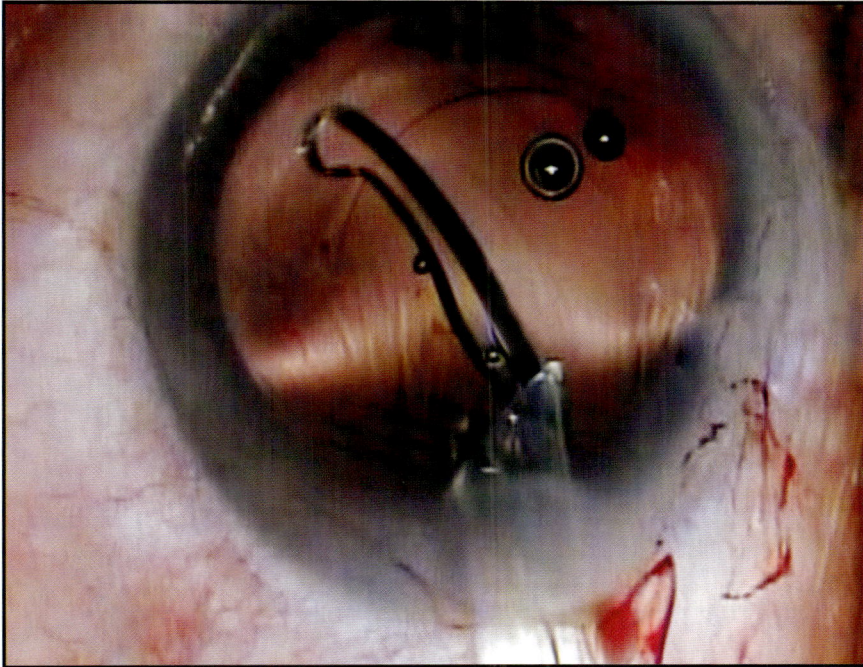

Fig. 20.8A: IOL being released into the bag loading hepatic undermeath the anterior capsule

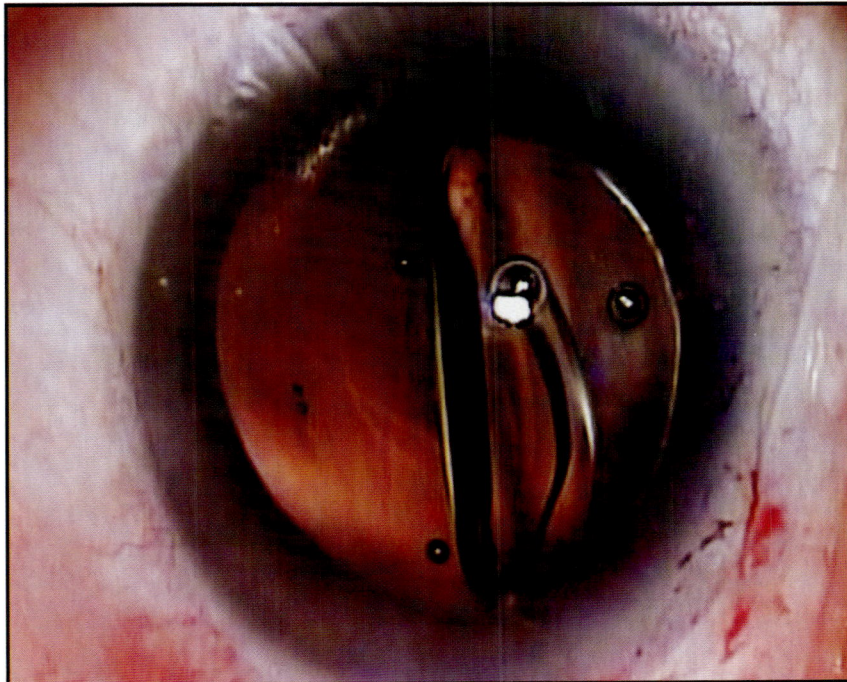

Fig. 20.8B: IOL released into the bag upper hepatic unfolded

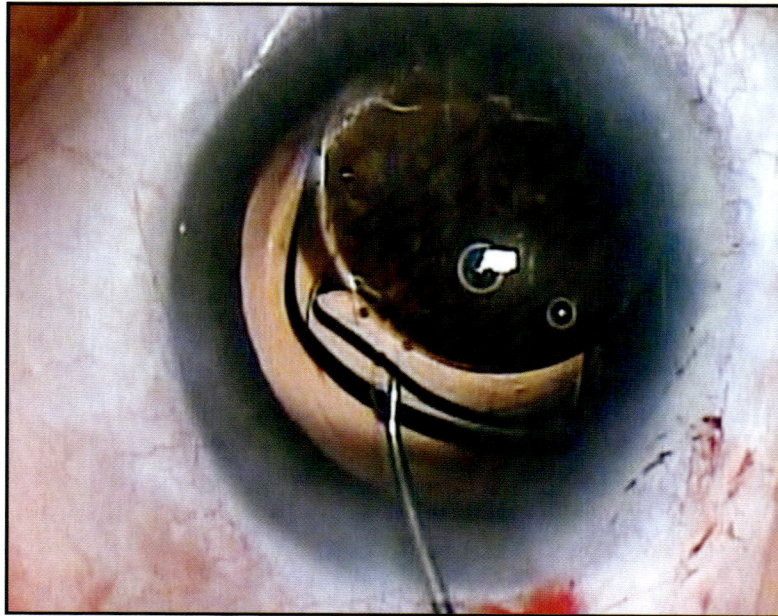

Fig. 20.8C: IOL is di aled in the bag

- The remaining viscoelastic present in the bag and the anterior chamber is aspirated

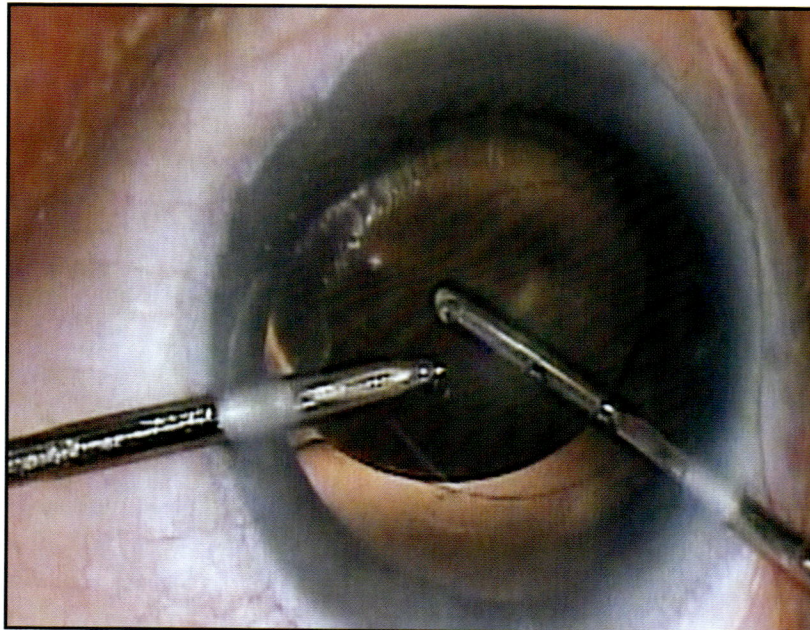

Fig. 20.9: Removal of the OVD at the end of surgery

- The wound is closed using mild cautery and subconjunctival antibiotic and steroids are given
- Side port is hydrated

Section

4

Surgery In Special Situations

21

Hard Cataract

Difficulties in a Hard Cataract

- Poor visibility of red reflex.
- *Capsular changes:* Atrophic capsule is seen, resulting in posterior capsular dehiscence and zonular dialysis. Some cases present with capsulo-cortical or capsulo-nuclear adhesions, which makes the process of nuclear rotation difficult.
- Large, hard and fibrous lens demands high and prolonged phaco power.

Management

Plan

1. CCC must be larger than usual.
2. Hydrodissection must be gentle to avoid the complication of posterior capsular rent.
3. Hydrodelineation will not be possible.
4. Phaco machine –
   - Select high end machine
   - Burst mode is preferable
   - Sharp tip is preferable.
5. Avoid forcible nuclear rotation.

Procedure

Management of Nucleus

Sculpting: It is essential to create a space in the center of the nucleus. This space is necessary for manipulation of lens fragments , phaco tip and chopper. If available, Kelman tip is advisable.

- 45° tip is used for sculpting and trenching
- 30° tip is used for fragment management.

My Choice of Procedure

1. I take 30° tip in the entire procedure
2. Entry wound is a little larger than the usual to allow some leakage which avoids incisional burns.
3. I always prefer to use a combination of dispersive and cohesive viscoelastics which is not only economical but also serves these dual purpose of endothelial protection and maintenance of AC (so that phaco power is delivered away from endothelium). e.g; Methyl cellulose with Viscoat, HPMC with Viscoat.

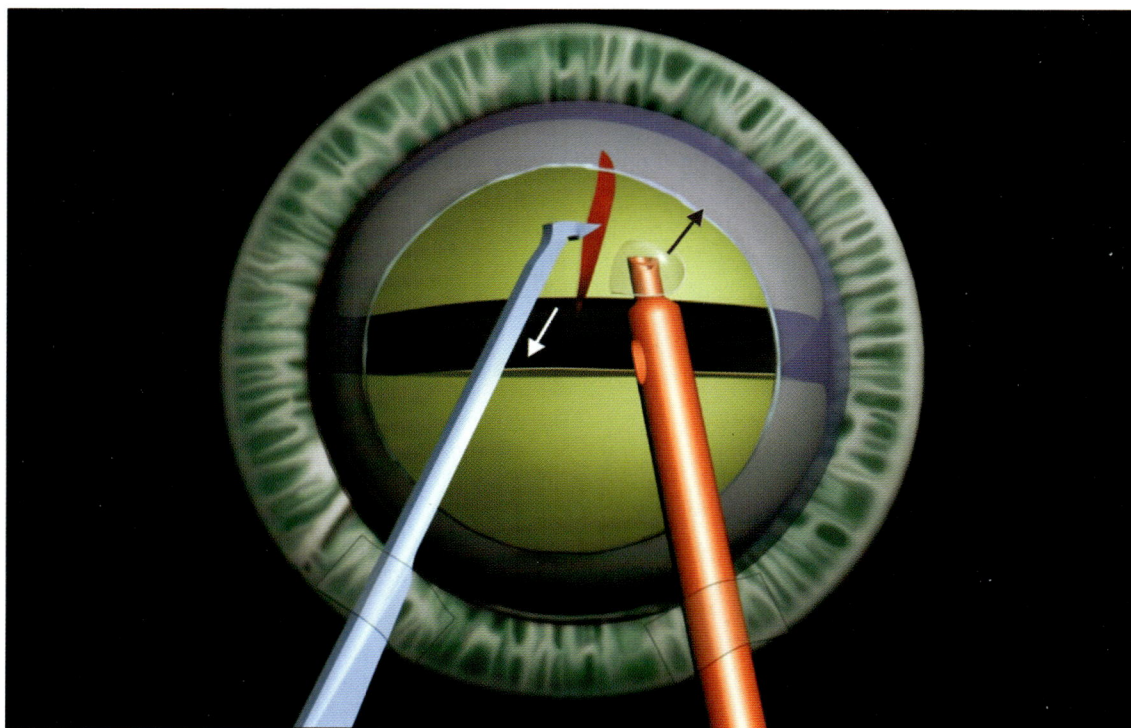

Fig. 21.1A: Trenching is done in one direction and nucleus is rotated with a chopper

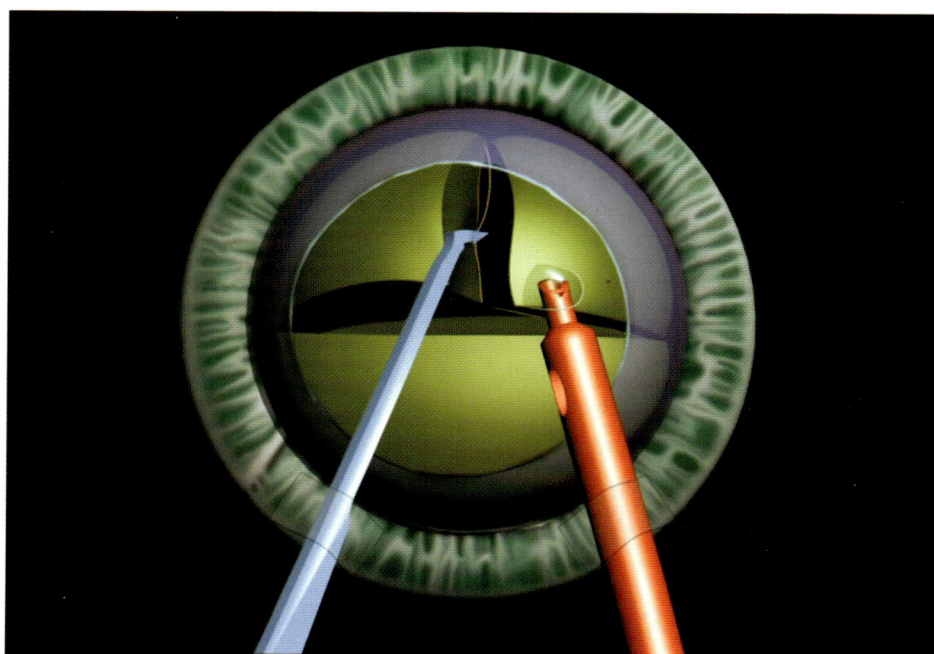

Fig. 21.1B: Trenching is done in the other direction to widen the groove with a chopper

4. Initial sculpting is done with Phaco I mode (80-20-20).The sculpting is useful
   - Create space
   - To debulk central hard core
   - To weaken the spine of the nucleus.

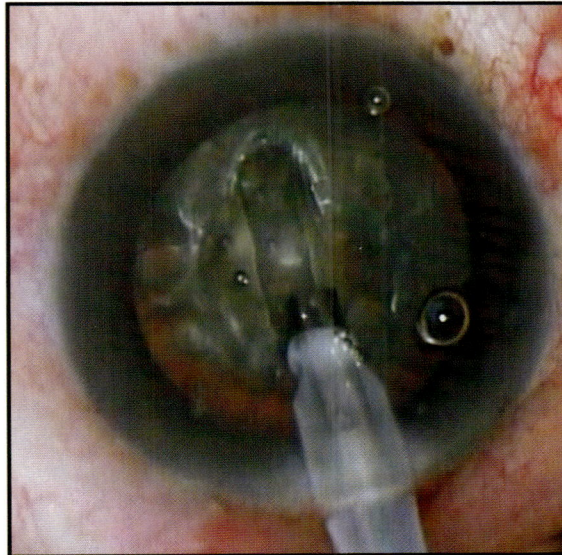

Fig. 21.1C: Trenching is done in the other direction

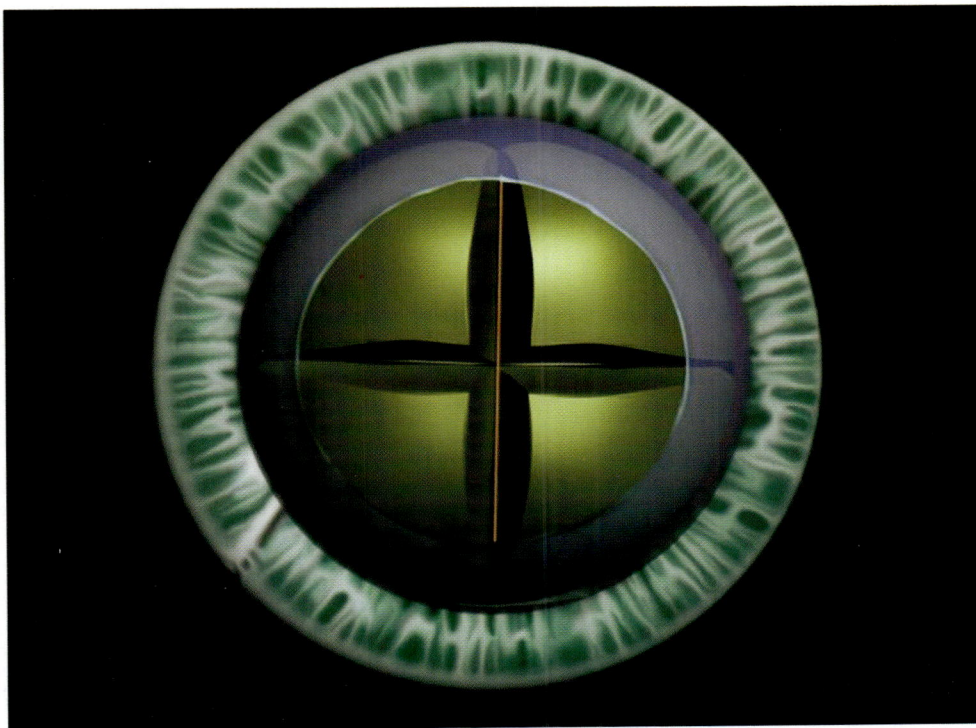

Fig. 21.1D: Four quardrant trenching is done

5. Next I switch to Phaco III (Burst mode 100%,25 cc,300 mm Hg) where lateral separation of the nucleus is done. Care is taken to separate the entire fragment separating even the small bridges of fibrous tissue.

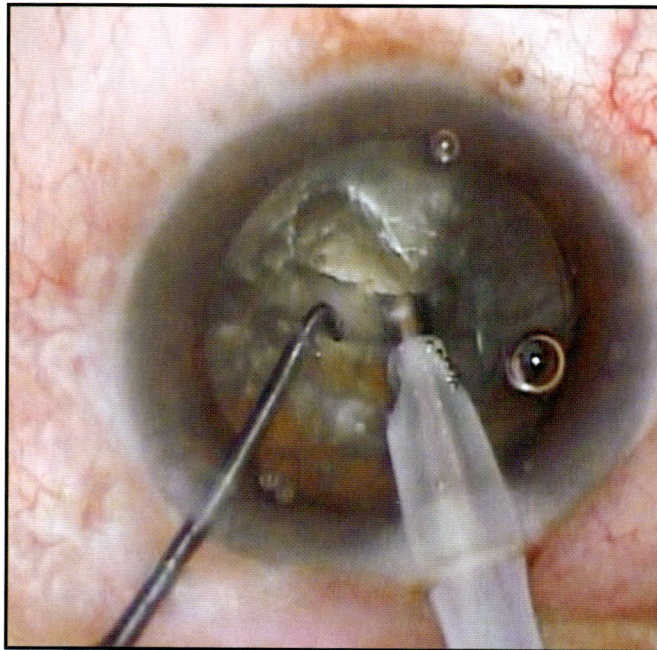

Fig. 21.1E: Quardrants are removed one by one in phaco II mode

6. I prefer to use the vertical chopper (tip and edges are sharp)

7. I divide the fragments into multiple pieces of smallest possible dimensions to reduce the phaco power needed. This exercise requires high levels of skill and patience.

8. These small fragments are easily emulsified using Phaco IV (high aspiration with 30 % of burst. It is preferable to do all the steps in the bag. Whenever the surgeon is not comfortable it is preferable to convert into SICS.

Some instances where the surgeon might have to convert to SICS are:

1. Prolonged Phaco
2. Inefficient Phaco
3. Zonular dialysis
4. Small PC rent.

22

Pediatric Cataract

Cataract Surgery in Children is a Challenging Exercise

Surgery should be performed by highly experienced surgeons, preferably those who are devoted to Pediatric services. It is not similar to surgery performed in adults.

Problems

- IOL Power calculation problems (refer chapter 5)
  1. Non co-operation
  2. Rapid change of IOL power with growth
- Shallow AC
- Highly elastic capsule
- Low scleral rigidity
- Pronounced post-operative inflammatory response
- Associated abnormalities of the eye
- Early and greater incidence of posterior capsular opacification
- Highly prone for stimulus deprivation amblyopia.

Procedures

- **Age less than 1 year:**
  1. Modified lensectomy where the visual axis is cleared by removing the central anterior and posterior capsules along with the lens and anterior vitrectomy is performed.
  2. Peripheral rim of anterior and posterior capsule are retained for future lens implants.
  3. Till the time the IOL can be implanted, contact lens can be used in case of unilateral cataracts and aphakic glasses can be used for bilateral cataracts.

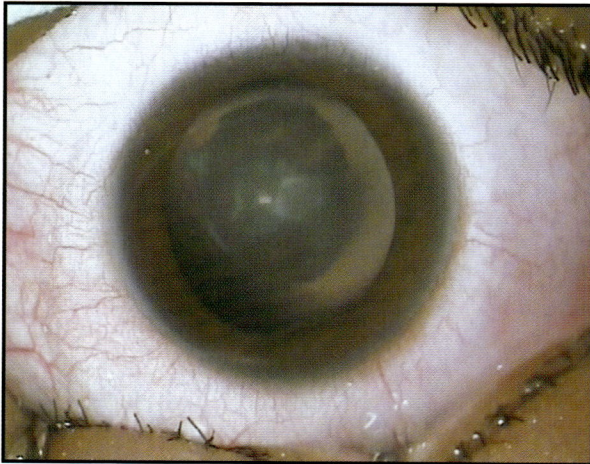

Fig. 22.1A: Pediatric cataract

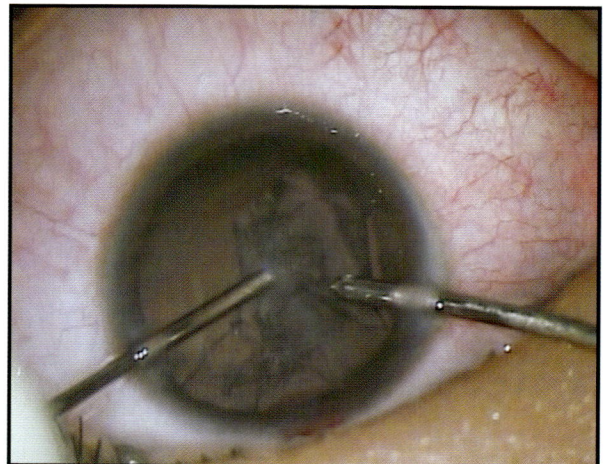

Fig. 22.1B: Aspiration of the lens matter using I and A

Age 1 to 5 years

1. Anterior CCC is done
2. Bimanual aspiration of lens matter is performed
3. Posterior CCC with anterior vitrectomy is performed
4. 3 piece hydrophobic IOL implantation is done.

Age more than 5 years

1. Phaco aspiration with single piece hydrophobic IOL
2. Yag capsulotomy whenever necessary.

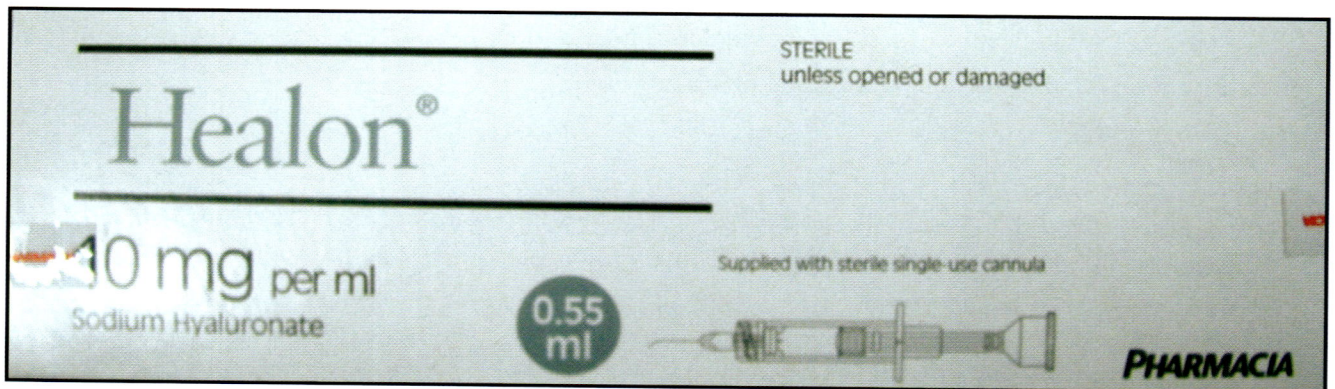

Fig. 22.2: Healon (high molecular weight viscoelastic)

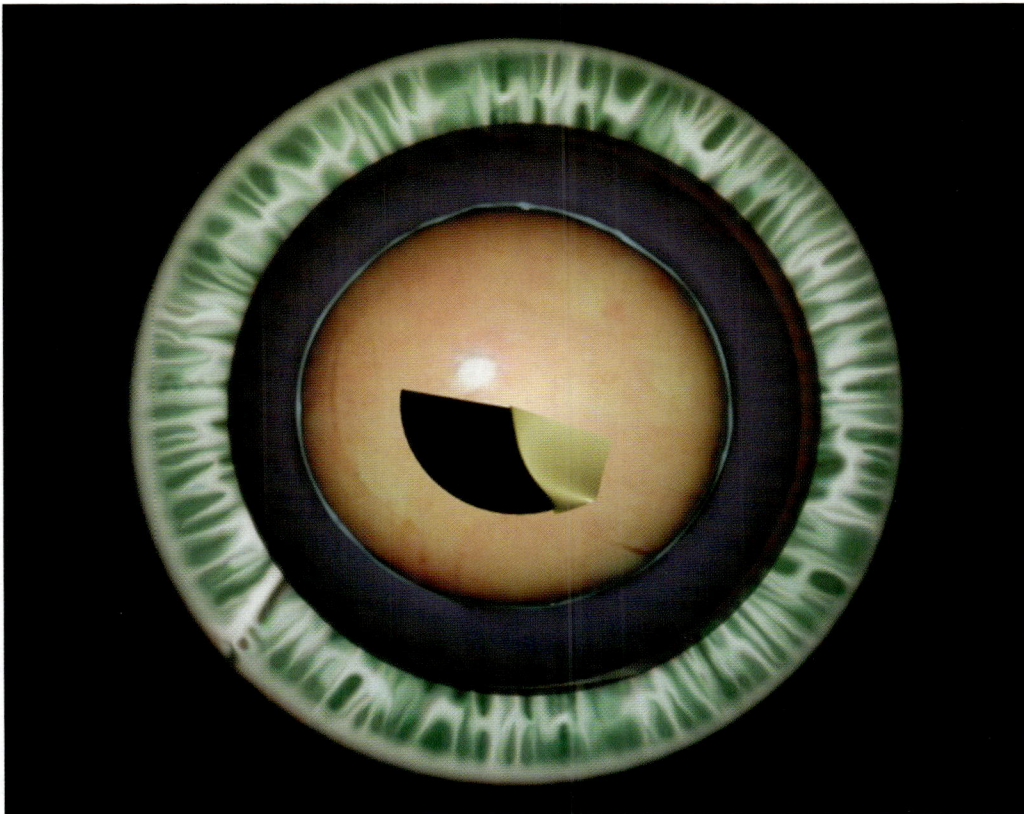

Fig. 22.3: Posterior capsulorhexis has to be done in cases of pediatric cataracts to avoid PCO

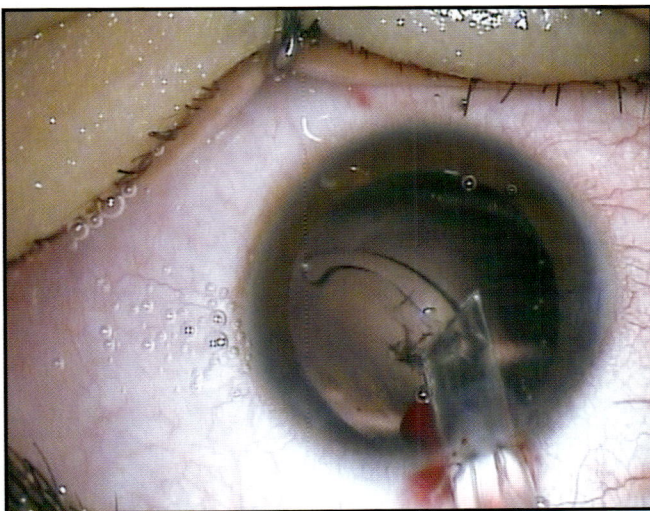

Fig. 22.4A: IOL insertion

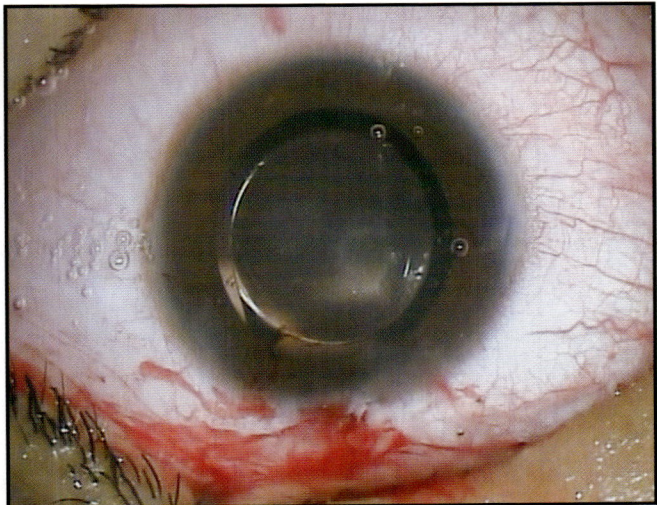

Fig. 22.4B: IOL in situ

I prefer to perform sclerocorneal tunnel incision even though there is a foldable lens implantation to avoid wound leaks and anterior synechiae formation because AC is shallow in small eyes and no suture will be required.

The usage of high molecular weight viscoelastic is advisable to maintain a deep anterior chamber.

The IOL power is calculated and 20% under correction is done. Post-operative residual correction is done using multifocal glasses.

Occlusion therapy is resorted to whenever necessary.

Fibrinoid reaction is common in the pediatric age group, especially in the new born. This is treated with intense topical steroids and mydriatics post-operatively.

23

Cataract and Glaucoma

Presentations
They may present as
- Cataract and glaucoma independent of each other
- Glaucoma induced cataract due to anti-glaucoma medications
- Cataract induced glaucoma (lens induced glaucoma)
- Pathological conditions that cause both glaucoma and cataract as in uveitis and the usage of steroids.

Treatment Options
- Cataract surgery only
- Combined surgery.

Cataract Surgery Alone
- Cataract surgery alone is indicated when glaucoma is well controlled with medical line of treatment
- When IOP is borderline with minimal or no glaucomatous changes.

Combined Surgery
- Combined surgery is resorted to when the above said conditions are not satisfied
- When patient is non compliant
- When the patient does not want to use medications after surgery.

Technique
Cataract surgery alone:
- Preoperative IOP reduction
- Management of miotic pupil
- Usage of CTR rings in pseudoexfoliation syndromes and subluxated lens.

Combined Procedures

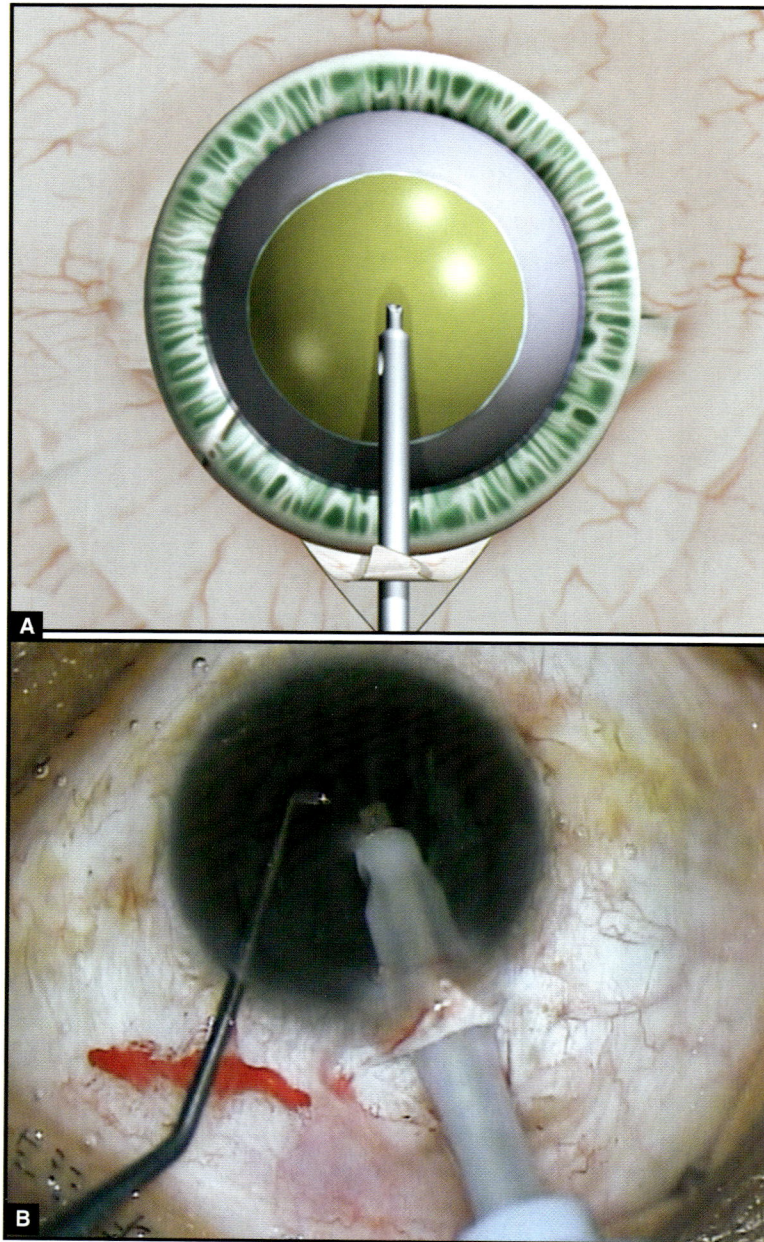

Figs 23.1A and B: Combined cataract surgery and trabeculectomy triangular scleral flap is taken

Phaco-Trabeculectomy/ SICS Trabeculectomy

Trabeculectomy and cataract are performed simultaneously usually from 12 O' clock area using either rigid PMMA 5.5 mm incision or 3 mm foldable lenses.

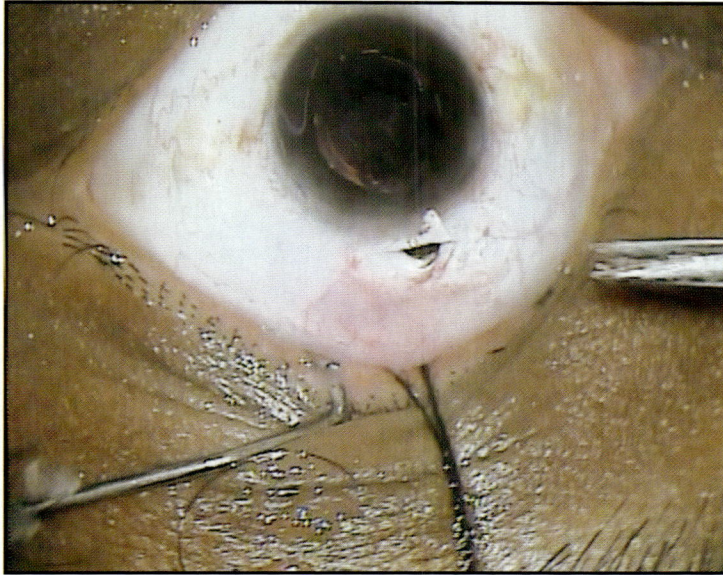

Fig. 23.1C: Trabeculectomy opening

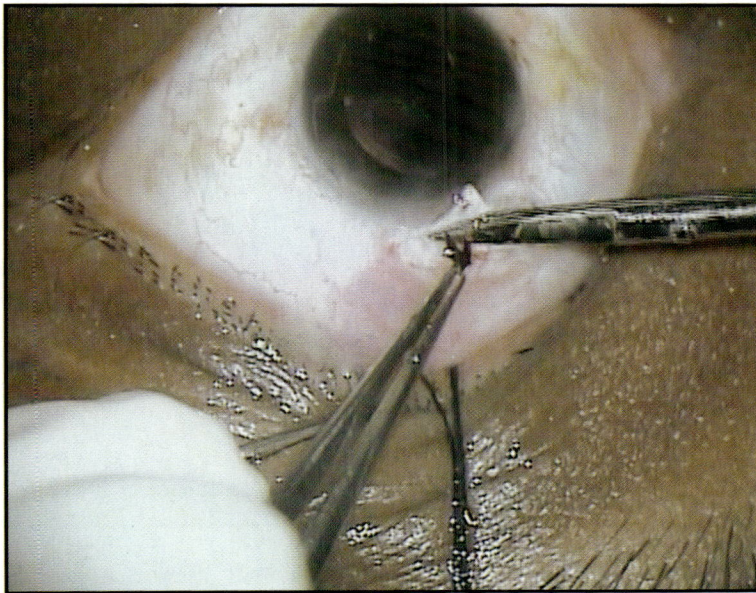

Fig. 23.1D: Iridectomy being done

• Anti-metabolites are added whenever indicated

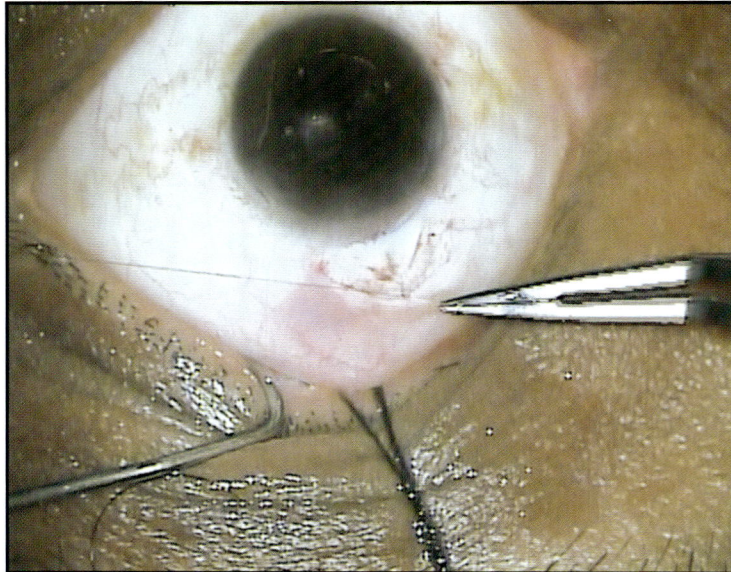

Fig. 23.1E: Scleral flap is sutured back with a single suture using 10 O' nylon

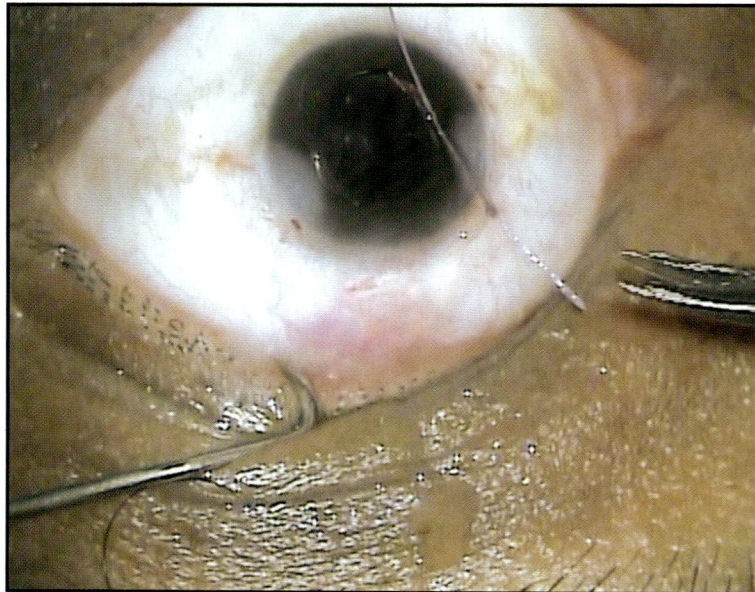

Fig. 23.1F: Conjunctival flap sutured with vicryl

Separate Sites

• Temporal clear corneal incision phaco with foldable IOL insertion is performed
• Later the surgeon shifts to 12 O' clock position
• Limbal based flap is raised and trabeculectomy is performed
• Conjunctiva is closed by continuous 8-0 vicryl suture.

In my experience, the inflammatory reaction and membrane formation is slightly higher in a combined surgery as compared to cataract surgery alone. Hence intra and post-operative intense steroid therapy and frequent follow ups of these patients is essential.

In the bag implantation is a must. If the patient is willing to continue antiglaucoma medication I prefer doing cataract surgery alone.

24

Posterior Polar Cataract

- Posterior polar cataracts are usually associated with 10% chances of posterior capsular rents during surgeries
- A preoperative diagnosis and proper planning will avoid vitreous loss and nuclear loss during surgery
- My preferred choice is CCC with Pre Chop technique where the size of CCC is neither too small nor too large
- Too small a CCC may result in difficulty in prolapsing the nucleus
- Too large a rhexis may result in inadequate IOL support
- Hydrodissection is to be avoided in these patients.

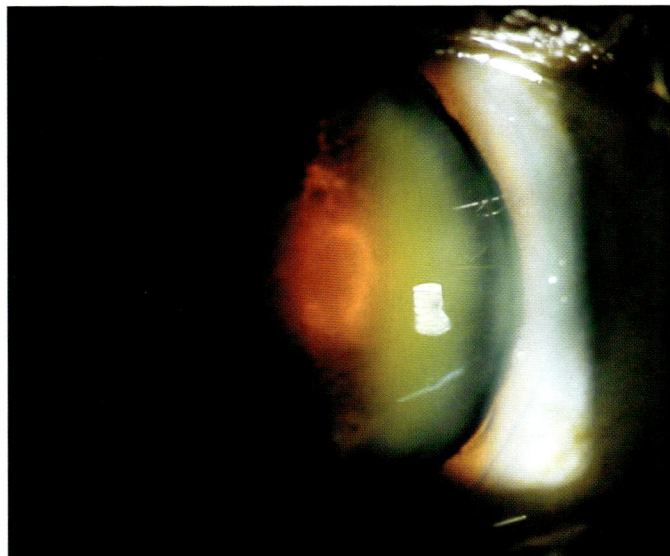

Fig. 24.1: Posterior polar cataract

Hydrodelineation

- Central groove is created with cystitome
- 26 gauge cannula with Balanced Salt Solution is inserted into this groove in center of nucleus and hydrodelineation is done from center to periphery (inside out). This exercise avoids accidental hydrodissection
- The same groove is used to weaken the spine of the nucleus so that the nucleus can be broken into 2 pieces during the hydroprocedure.

Phaco

- The 2 pieces are aspirated by phaco as most of the times 90% of the lens is clear and soft in posterior polar cataract
- The remaining epinucleus acts as a cushion and avoids Posterior Capsular Rent
- The remaining epinucleus and cortical removal is done in a centripetal fashion leaving the central plaque till the end
- At this stage, the IOL is implanted
- As a last step, an attempt is made to remove the plaque and polish the capsule
- Some of the cases may end in small PC rents without vitreous loss and the post-operative results are good.

25

Cataract in Myopia

Preoperative Evaluation

- Appropriate biometry using Holladay's formula
- B-scan to identify the presence and location of staphyloma if any
- Selection of appropriate IOL. I prefer to use hydrophobic acrylic (Acrys of IOL) which has a large optic of 6 mm with adhesive surface which sticks to the capsule and a square edge which will prevent post-operative posterior capsular opacification and lessens the induced astigmatism.

Anesthesia

- I prefer to use topical anesthesia
- If the patient is unco-operative, modified topical or subtenon's injection can be used
- If the patient is still unco-operative general anesthesia is preferred
- I avoid peribulbar and retrobulbar anesthesia in high myopic eyes as there is more chance of trauma to globe and retina.

Procedure

Incision: Shorter, temporal tunnel (clear corneal) is preferred.

Capsulorhexis: A normal capsulorhexis is done. Care should be taken that rhexis opening is well centered to avoid posterior capsular opacification.

Hydrodissection

1. If the nucleus is soft and small as in clear lens extraction ,it is preferable to prolapse the nucleus into anterior chamber during hydrodissection.
2. If it is large and hard, gentle multipoint dissection and free rotation of the nucleus in the capsular bag is attempted.

Phaco

Usually the chamber is very deep. To avoid excessive depth, decrease the height of the bottle and the flow rate.

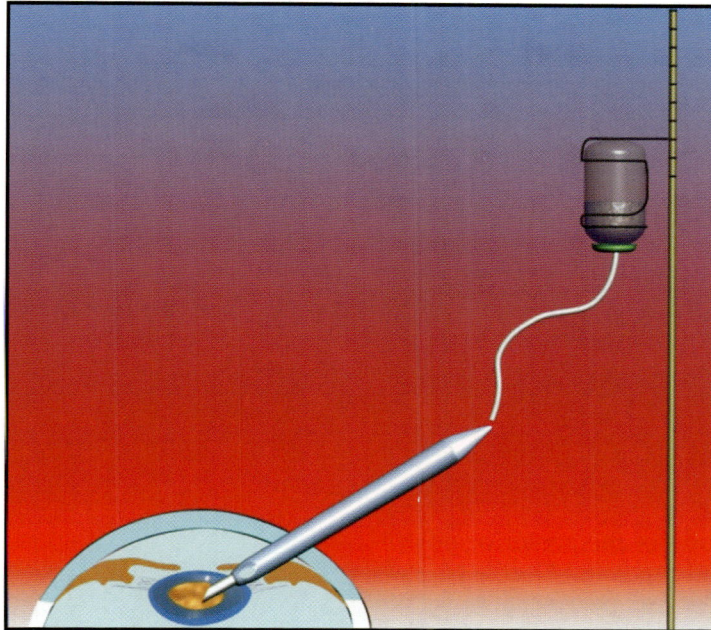

Fig. 25.1: When bottle height is decreased AC becomes shallow

2. The nucleus is disproportionately harder than it's color may suggest (underestimated). Hence gentle high power low aspiration phaco is essential.
3. Beware of weak zonules during Phaco and nuclear manipulation.

Irrigation and Aspiration

To delay posterior capsular opacification, bimanual irrigation and aspiration with thorough polishing of the capsule is essential.

In conclusion, the degree of satisfaction expressed by a myopic patient after the removal of the cataractous /clear lens is high as he will be independent of spectacles. Care should be taken to manage the deep seated cataract with weak zonules.

26

Cataract in Uveitis

Why Surgery is Needed?

1. To improve vision
2. To improve visualization of the posterior pole.

When?

- No surgery must be attempted in the presence of active inflammation as evidenced by the presence of congestion, keratic precipitates or hypopyon
- Surgery is attempted only when inflammation subsides and the eye is quiet for a period of three months
- Prior to surgery, preoperative B-scan is mandatory to rule out Retinal detachment .

Steroids

- Preoperative: 1 week prior to surgery, topical steroids with mydriatics and systemic steroids are to be started
- Intraoperative: On table depot preparation is to be given (Sub Tenon's)
- Post-operative: Systemic as well as intense topical steroids are to be given.

Procedures

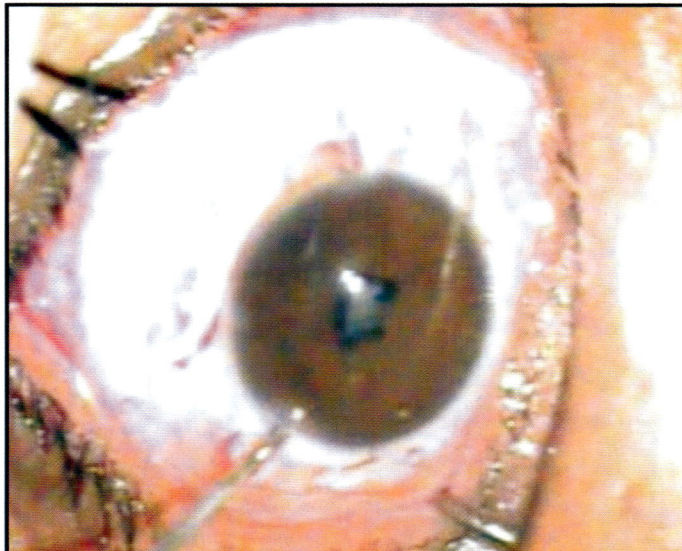

Fig. 26.1A: Complicated cataract (post inflamatory) pupil is miotic due to synechiae

Management of Pupil

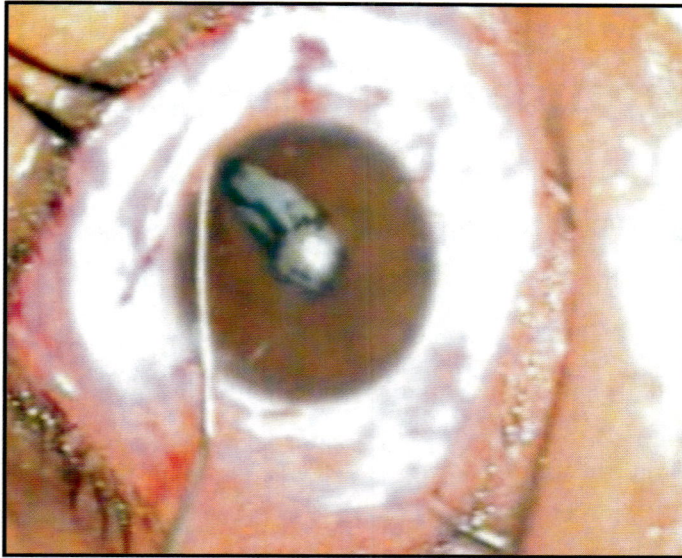

Fig. 26.1B: Syneicholysis

- Viscosynechiolysis: Majority of cases can be managed
- Pupil can be mechanically manipulated using "Y" dialer
- If there is a fibrotic membrane underneath the iris, it can be peeled off or dissected
- In difficult cases iris retractors can be used.

Phaco

- Large CCC is a must. Small CCC may result in post-operative phimosis and irido capsular adhesions
- Can opener technique commonly causes pupillary capture
- Gentle maneuvres are advised to avoid injury to iris or capsule.

Heparin: Intra cameral heparin (10 IU/ml) is added in the irrigating bottle to reduce post-operative inflammation.

IOL: Heparin or fluorine surface modified IOL is preferred .

Vitrectomy: If there is considerable debris in the vitreous or persistent macular edema, combined vitrectomy and cataract surgery will help the patient .

Summary: Perioperative steroids, Heparin and in the bag Heparin modified IOL will help these patients.

28

Subluxated Lens

Causes

- Trauma
- During surgery
- Pseudoexfoliation
- Marfan's syndrome

Preoperative Evaluation

Slit-Lamp Examination

1. Irregular AC depth
2. Vitreous in AC
3. Phacodonesis
4. Wrinkles on anterior capsule

Indirect Ophthalmoscopy: Lens margin can be seen.

Gonioscopy: Look for angle recession secondary to glaucoma.

B-scan: To check for posterior capsular integrity.

Management

Zonular dehiscence:
Less than 45° - PCIOL is placed in the bag or sulcus
Less than 180° - Capsular tension ring(CTR)
More than 180° - Cionni ring (Modified CTR) or scleral fixated IOL

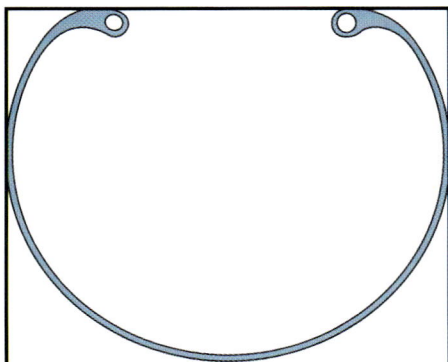

Fig. 28.1A: Capsular tension ring (CTR)

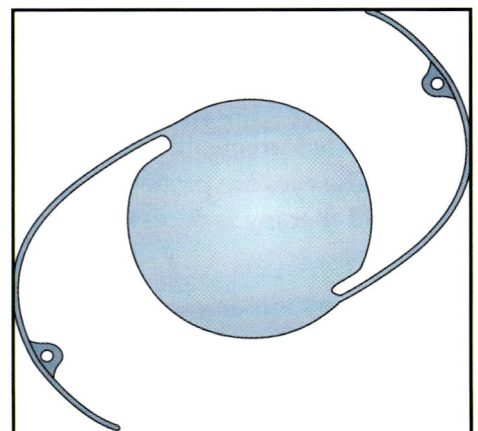

Fig. 28.1B: Scleral fixation IOL

Operative Pearls

1. Large capsulorhexis
2. Insert CTR ring away from dehiscence
3. Insert with forceps/shooter
4. 8-0 vicryl suture are applied to one of the eye of CTR ring to ensure retrieval of the ring in case of a sinkage
5. SICS/Phaco
6. Gentle chopping of nucleus is done

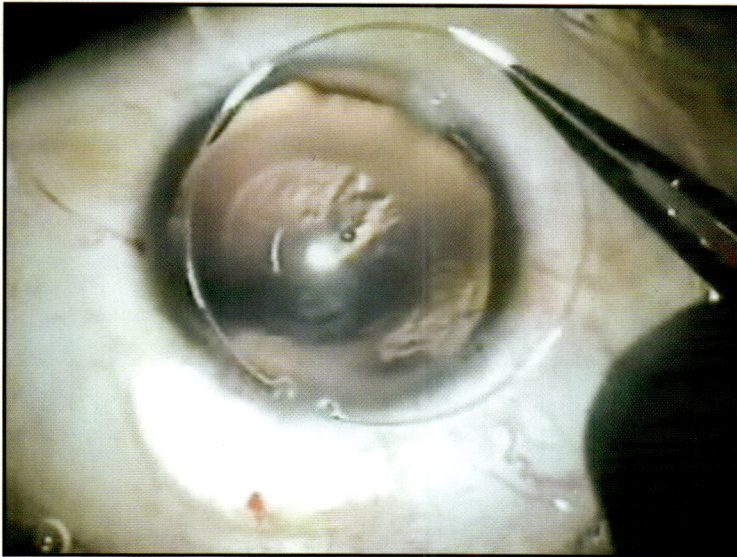

Fig. 28.1C: CTR should be introduced into the capsular bag immediately after performing a rhexis

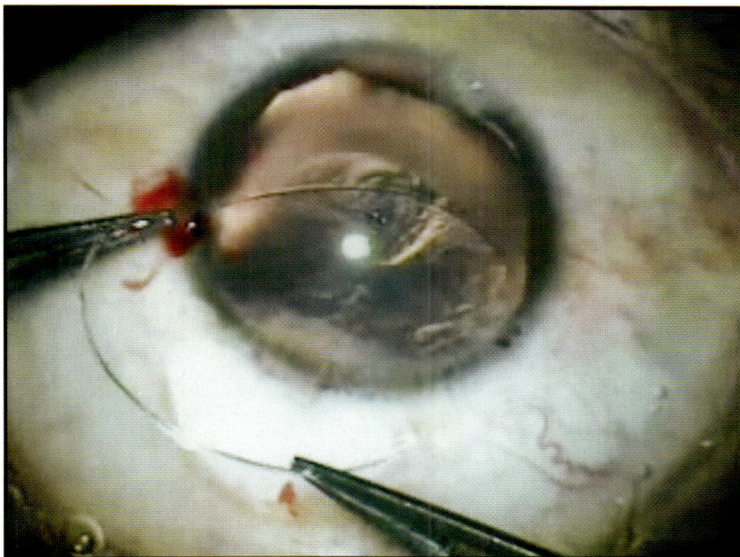

Fig. 28.1D: CTR being passed under the rhexis

Advantages of CTR Ring

- It is a better alternative to anterior chamber lens or scleral fixated lens
- It is cost effective
- The technique is not very difficult to learn
  The outcome in most of the cases is good despite difficult conditions of operation .

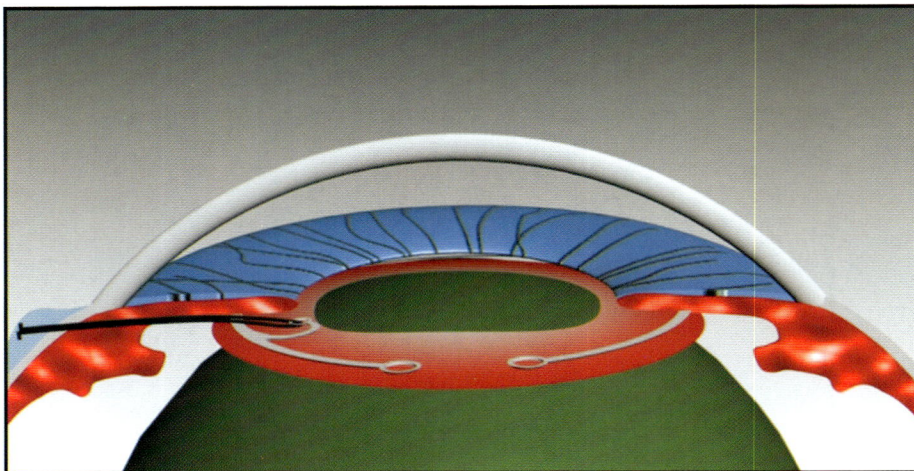

Fig. 28.1E: CTR in position

29

Miotic Pupil

Causes

1. Senile miosis
2. Pseudoexfoliation
3. Diabetes mellitus
4. Posterior uveitis
5. Glaucoma therapy
6. Trauma
7. Idiopathic

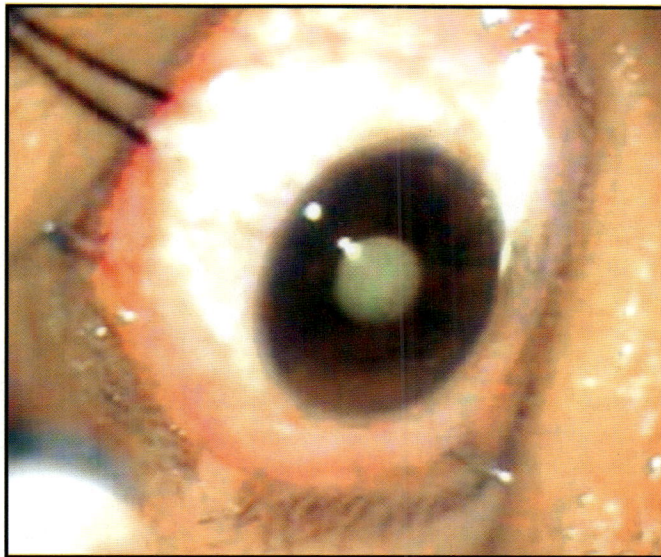

Fig. 29.1: Mature cataract with miotic pupil

If the pupil had been dilated in the previous 24 hours, the dilatation response to subsequent applications of topical mydriatics might not be optimal due to the phenomenon of pupillary fatigue.

In such cases, it is advisable to postpone the case by a day to allow for the recovery from this episode of fatigue.

Management

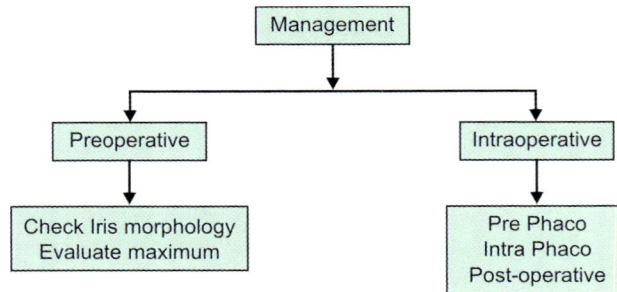

Pre phaco management:
- Adrenaline in the bottle
- Visco mydriasis
- Synechiolysis
- Iris surgery.

Iris Surgery

1. Partial sphincterotomy
2. Mid iris iridectomy
3. Inferior sphincterotomy
4. Multiple sphincterotomies

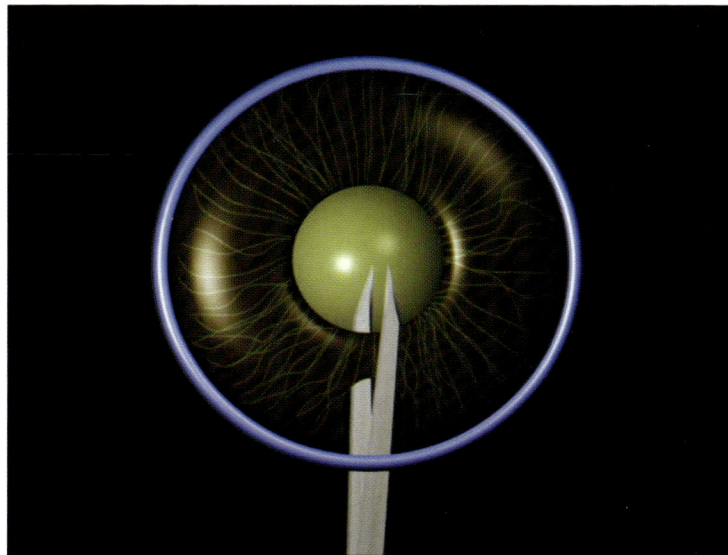

Fig. 29.2: Mid iris iridectomy

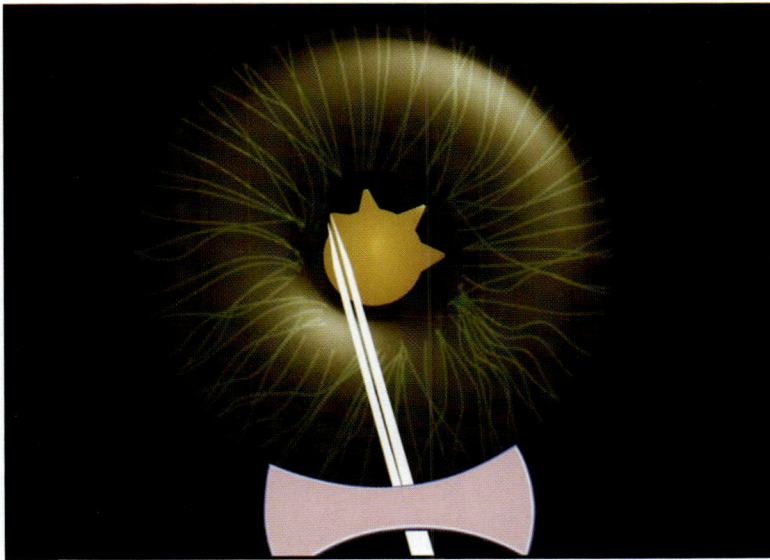

Fig. 29.3: Multiple sphincterotomies

Manipulation of Pupil

1. Visco mydriasis (Healon 5)
2. Pupillary stretch
3. Beehler speculum
4. Iris hooks
5. Iris protector ring
6. Pupil ring expander.

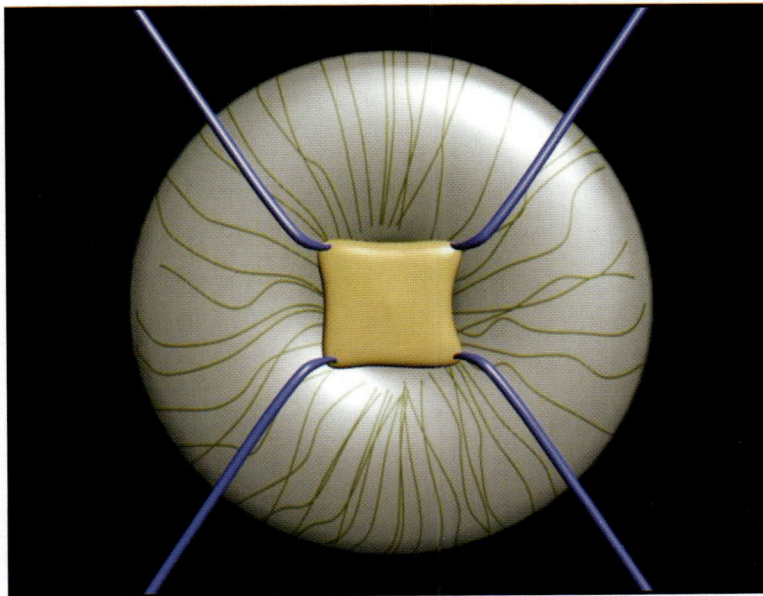

Fig. 29.4: Dilating the pupil using iris hooks

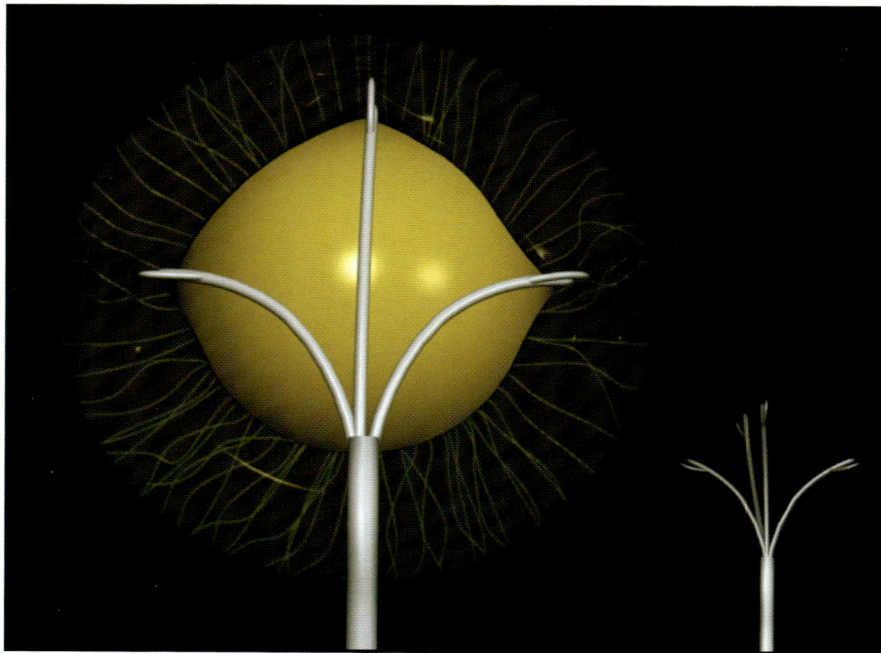

Fig. 29.5: Dilatation of pupil using Bheeler's speculum

Some of these procedures cause dilatation at the cost of sphincter dysfunction. However, the sphincter dysfunction is preferable to posterior capsular rent, vitreous loss and their subsequent complications.

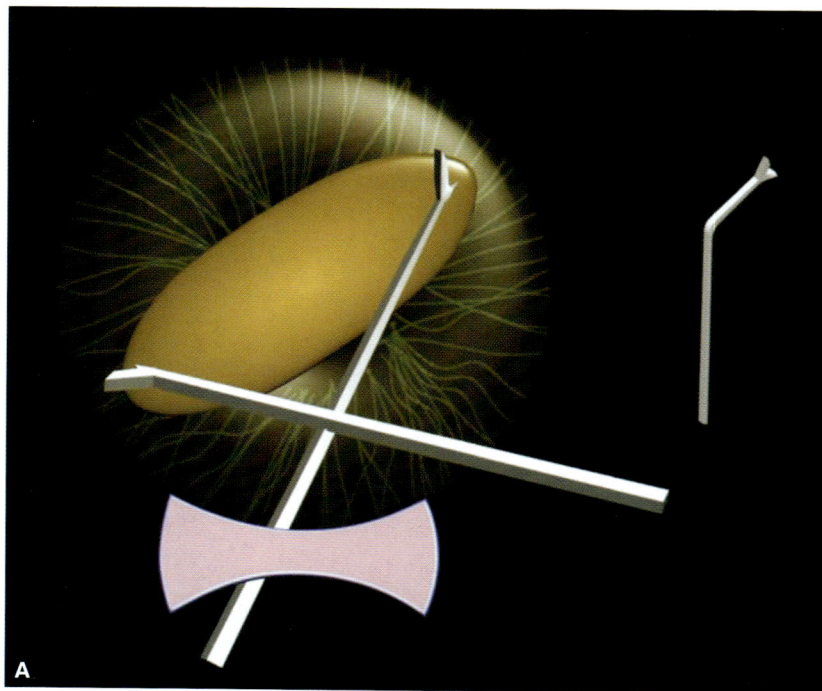

Fig. 29.6A: Dilatation the pupil using 'Y' pushers in cross action

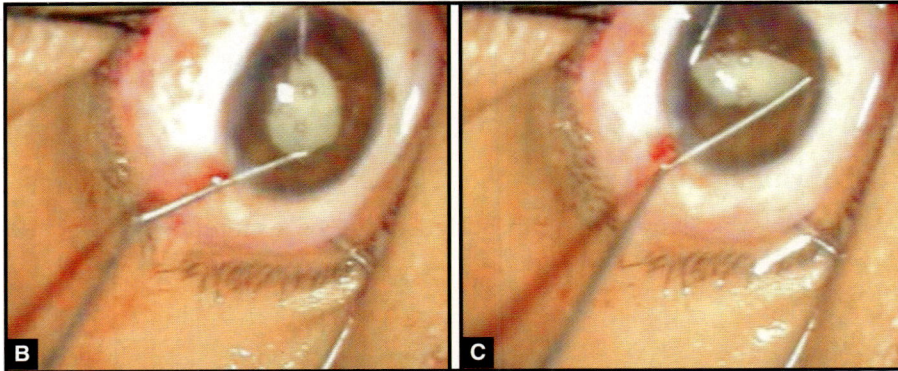

Figs 29.7B and C: Dilating the pupil using 'Y' pushers

Intra Phaco Management

- CCC under the iris, hence larger than the pupillary size
- Phaco chop technique is used.
  1. Hydro dis-section is done to enable nuclear rotation
  2. Deep, short narrow groove is created
  3. Kelman tip is used
  4. Chopping is performed *in situ*
  5. Lateral separation of the fragments is done.

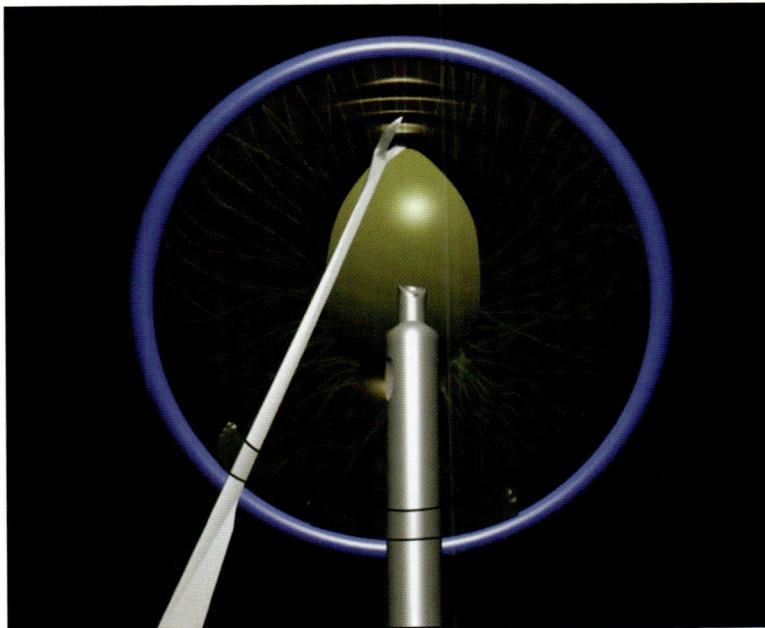

Fig. 29.7: Intraoperative (phaco) iris retaction

- Bimanual irrigation aspiration is used
- Intraoperative retraction of Iris
- Single piece foldable IOL
- Ensure miosis at the end of the procedure .

Post-operative Phaco Management

- More aggressive use of topical steroids with added usage of systemic steroids if necessary to control inflammation.
- More frequent follow-ups.

30

Microincision Phacoemulsification or Bimanual Phaco or Phaconit

The incision size in conventional phaco is 2.5-3 mm. The incision size is limited by the size of the tip and the IOL. To reduce the size of the incision the infusion sleeve has to be separated from the phaco tip. The IOL should be designed so that it can be introduced through smaller incisions.

COLD PHACOEMULSIFICATION

Ultrasonic energy used to emulsify the nucleus raises the temperature at the tip of the phaco probe. This causes damage to the endothelial cells (almost 30%) and incisional burns.

Several new systems can perform cold phacoemulsification.They are:

1. *Laser Based:*

   Paradigm Photon; Aesculap-Meditec Phacolase; Premier Centauri; ARC Dodick; Adiago Wavelight

   These systems use laser to destroy nuclear material. They are safe and effective. But they can be used only for soft nuclei.

2. *Water Method:*

   Alcon Aqualase

   This system uses pulsed warm balanced salt solution to lyse the nucleus. This is useful for soft nuclei at the present. No ultrasonic energy is used in this procedure. Hence there is minimal damage to ocular tissues.

3. *Sonic System:*

   STAAR sonic system

   The operating frequency is in the sonic rather than ultrasonic range .It is between 40-400 Hz .In contrast to ultrasonic tip motion the sonic tip moves back and forth without changing its dimensional length thereby avoiding frictional heat. It does not generate cavitational effects. Thus fragmentation occurs rather than emulsification or vaporization occurs.

4. *Ultrasonic Pulsed Phacoemulsification:*

   Oertli LMP; Neosonix Alcon; White Star Allergan

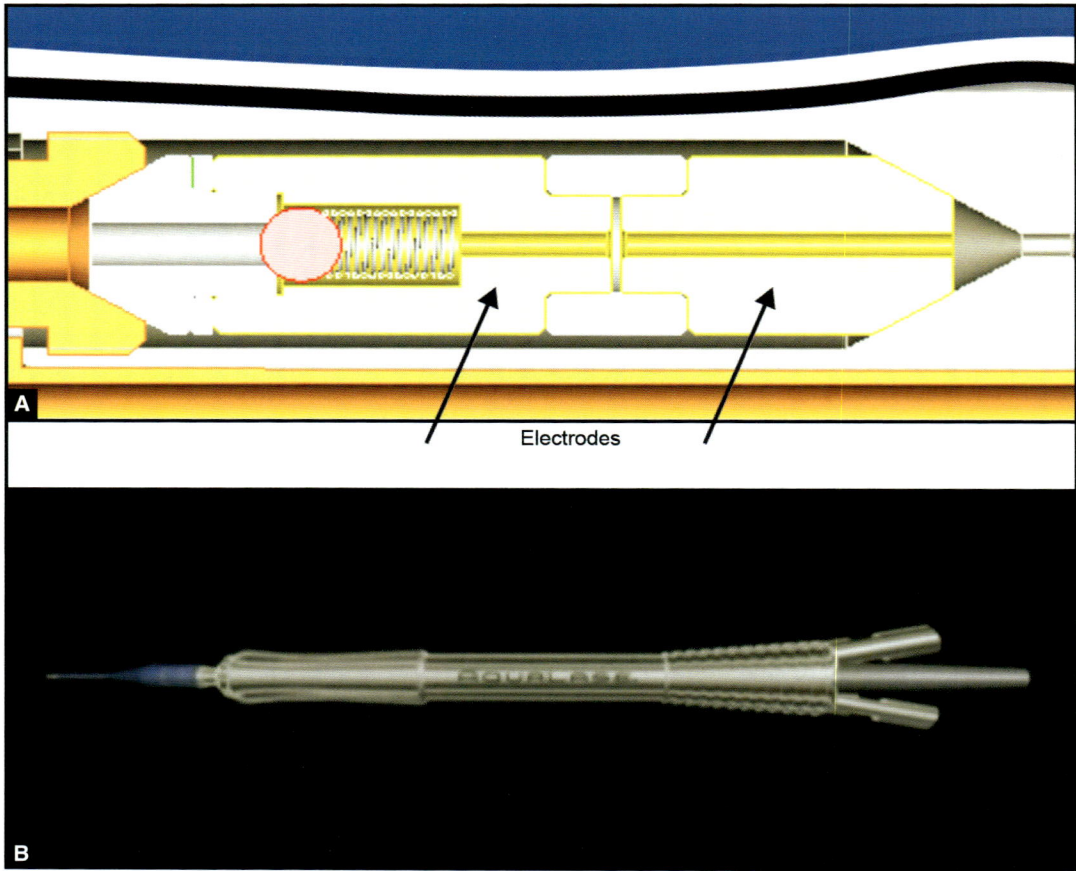

Electrodes

Figs 30.1A and B: Aqualase phaco probe

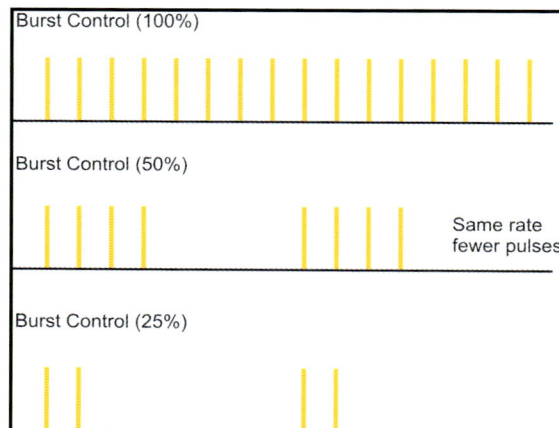

Burst Control (100%)

Burst Control (50%)

Same rate fewer pulses

Burst Control (25%)

Fig. 30.2: 100% energy is released continuously at regular intervals 50% energy is released in on phase (50%) and off phase (50%) no energy is released and cooling occurs 25% energy is released in on phase (25%) and off phase (75%)

Pulse technology is a software modification that allows extremely short bursts of ultrasonic energy. (ON-OFF). Energy is released in phase ON in a reduced percentage (up to 20%). So it is possible to prolong OFF phase which cools the tip. This decreases wound heat build up with retained efficiency of continuous ultrasonics. Thereby there is use of less energy and causes less corneal damage.

Preventing tip heating implies reduced incision width as we can use a normal tip without its irrigating sleeve. Incision size can be reduced to less than 3 mm, 0.9 mm (if 20G is used).

Ozil

This is also called torsional phaco. The ultrasound tip will have a torsional movement with angulaton. The advantage of this is no repulsion of nuclear fragments and thus efficient delivery of energy there by reducing the endothelial damage and wound burns. As to and fro movement is not there incidence of wound burns is minimal.The ideal procedure is to keep in the linear mode with 45° tip which helps in efficient removal of nucleus.

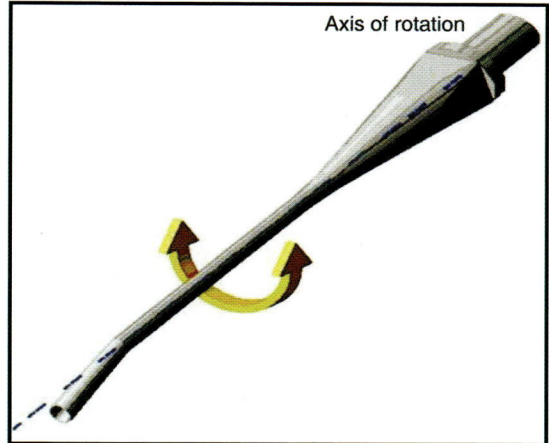

Fig. 30.3: Ozil (torsional phaco)

CUSTOM CONTROL SOFTWARE

Bausch and Lomb, MILLENNIUM

The new software creates hyperpulse phaco (High frequency pulse, emulate continuous phaco) up to 120 pps with adjustable phaco duration and rest time (duty cycle). The software also provides waveform modulation to further enhance energy efficiency and fragment followability.

Hyperpulse settings are programmable and intraoperative modifications of settings can be done. Intraoperative change of mode is also possible.

It also has wave form modulation.

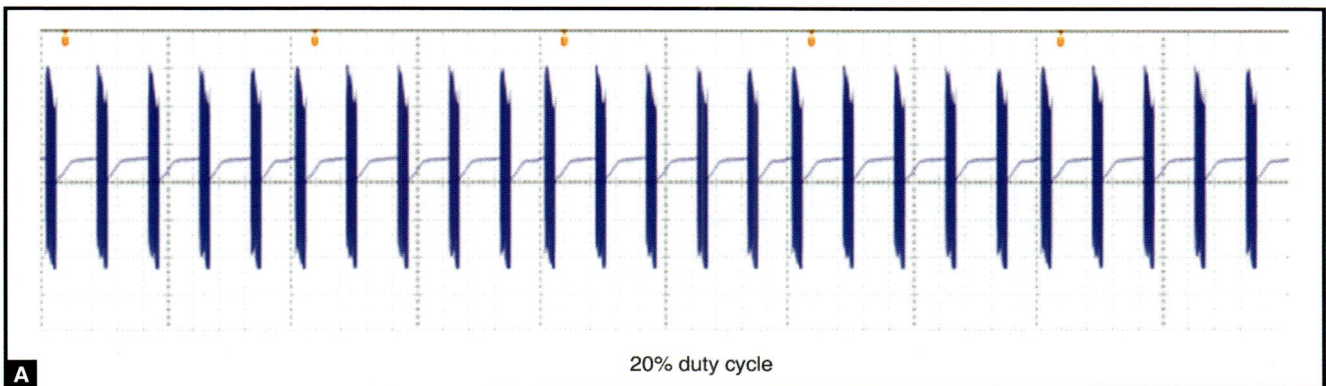

20% duty cycle

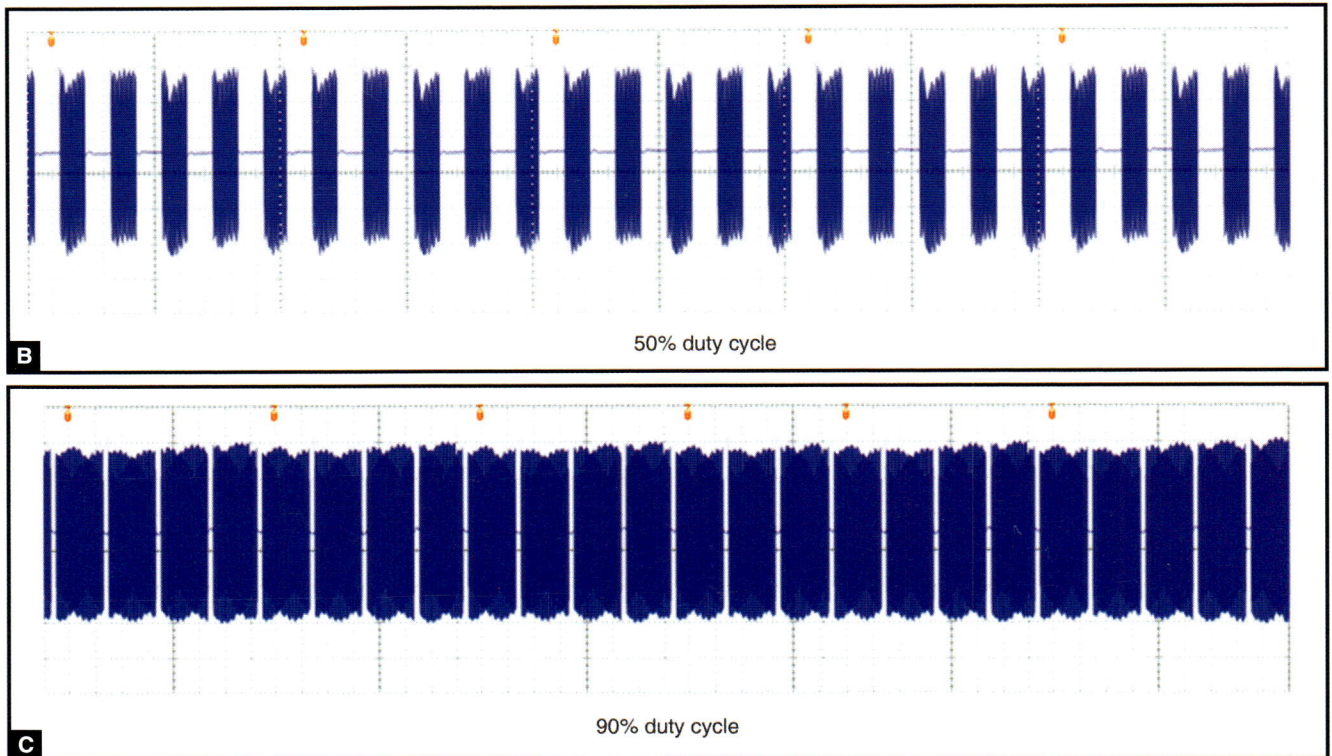

Figs 30.4A to C: 50 PPS, with different duty cycles (DC)

WAVEFORM PHACO MODULATION

Ramp up cycle (Wave): Phaco energy is delivered in the form of pocket of micropulses gradually increasing in power.

   Waveform Phaco provides better fragment followability during the gradually increasing phase.
   The Waveform further reduces heat generation to the minimum.

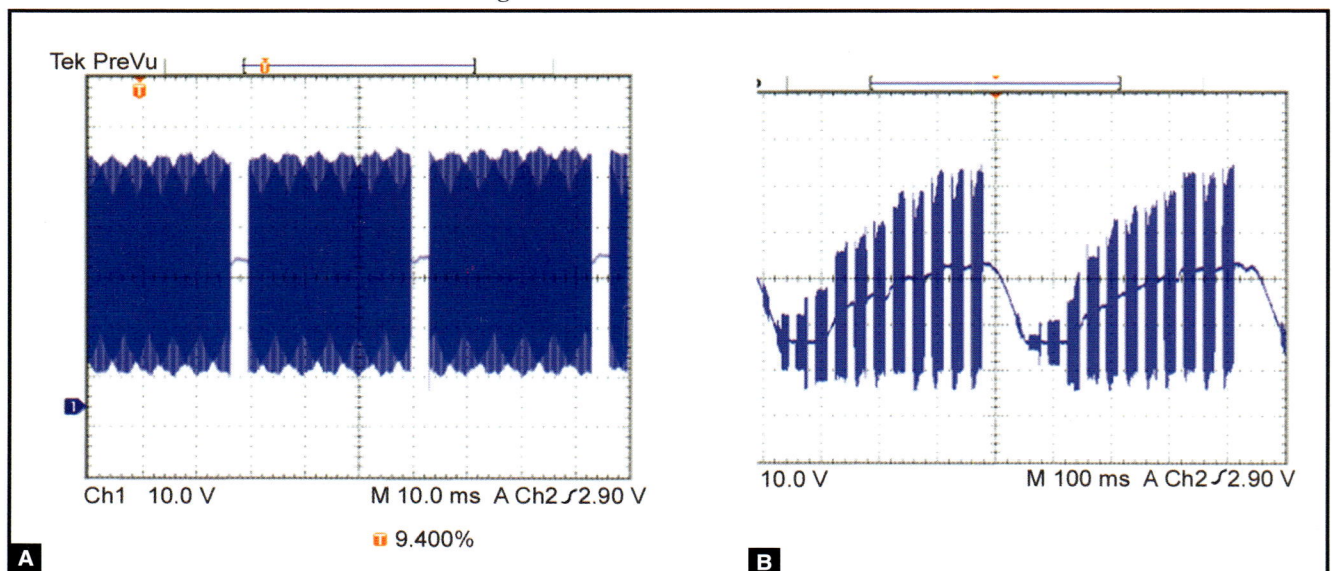

Figs 30.5A and B: Waveform phaco

Section
5

Complications

31

Complications of Cataract Surgery

INTRAOPERATIVE

Incision

a) **Depth:** Superficial—Leads to buttonholing.
        Stop and take the incision in a deeper plane
        Deep—It may injure the Iris and Ciliary body.

b) **Location:** Anterior incision—Insecure tunnel and needs
        Suturing the wound at the end of surgery
        Posterior incision—May cause premature entry, excessive bleeding from the wound and
         difficulty in prolapsing the nucleus.

c) **Length:** Long incision—Post-operative wound leak which needs suturing of the wound postoperative astigmatism
        Small incision—Difficulty in delivering the nucleus
        Leading to corneal endothelial damage.
        To avoid this it is always better enlarge the incision

d) **Side port incision:** There may be bleeding, iris prolapse
        Descemet's detachment
        Wound leak which needs a suture.

Descemet's detachment – may occur when entering into the anterior chamber from the main incision or side port incision.

A small detachment can be repositioned by injecting a tight air bubble into the anterior chamber at the end of surgery.

A big detachment needs a full thickness corneal suture.

Capsulotomy

In SICS incomplete capsulotomy' – causes difficulty in prolapsing the nucleus.

Rhexis: **Irregular rhexis** – the rhexis may run away to the Periphery

Too small: In SICS–difficult to prolapse the nucleus Into AC, radial cuts have to be made in the anterior capsule.
        In phaco–tear of rhexis margins may occur with the phaco tip difficulty in IOL insertion capsular stretch may cause posterior capsule folds.

Too large: In phaco prolapse of nuclear fragments into anterior chamber from the bag may occur
        Post-operative decentration of IOL.
        Posterior capsular opacification is more frequent if capsule margin is not overlapping the IOL.

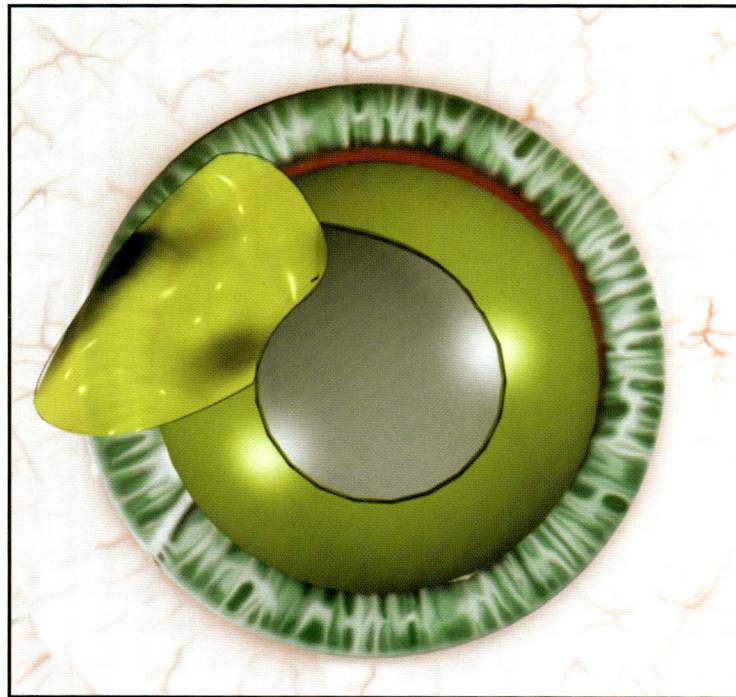

Fig. 31.1: Irregular capsulorhexis (the rhexis is moving away in to the periphery)

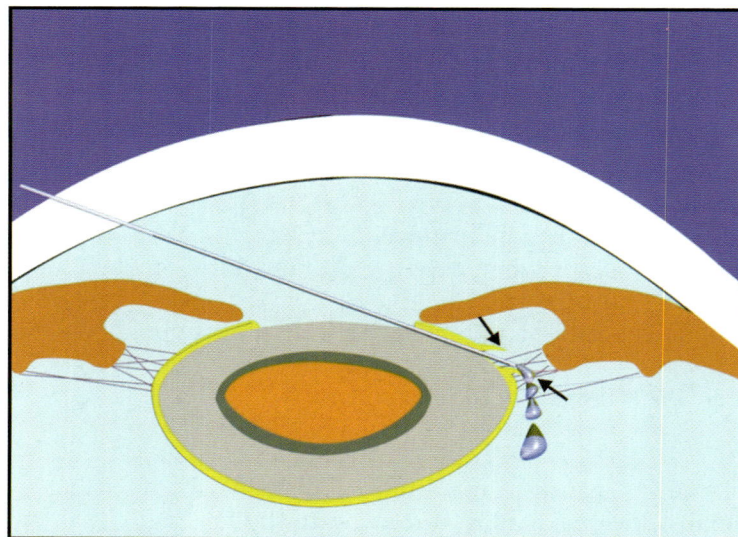

Fig. 31.2A: Zonnular damage during hydroprocedures

Hydroprocedures

Incomplete hydrodissection – causes difficulty in rotating the nucleus and damage to the zonule

Excessive fluid flow – can cause tear of rhexis

Damage to the zonule

PC rupture and loss of nucleus into vitreous

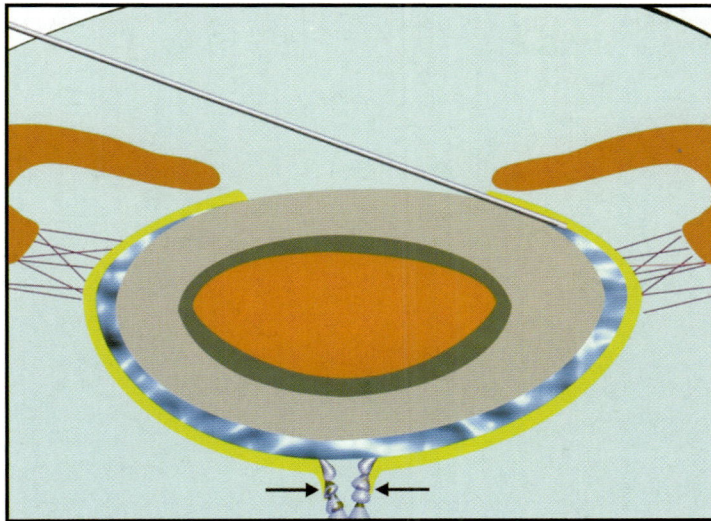

Fig. 31.2B: Posterior capsule rupture during hydroprocedures

Nucleus prolapse and delivery

In SICS, tearing of tunnel and corneal endothelial damage may occur. To avoid it, AC should be maintained deep by using fluid or viscoelastic.

Iridodialysis – repair has to be done.

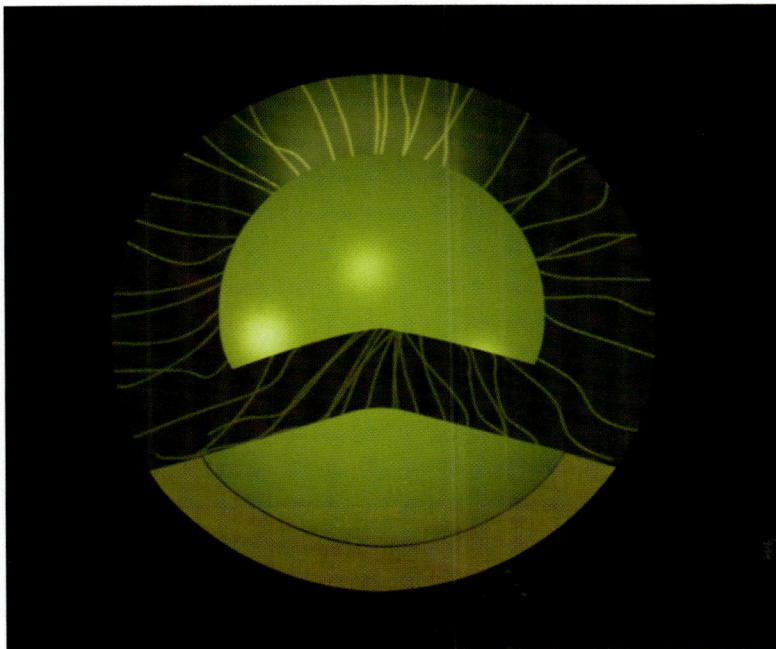

Fig. 31.3A: Iridodialysis–involving more than 3 O'clock hours

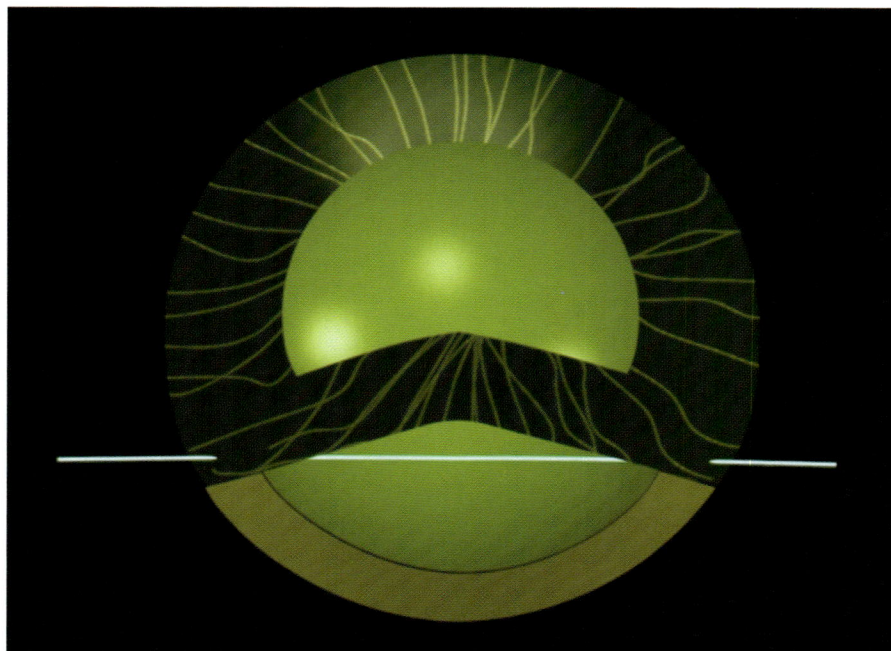

Fig. 31.3B: Iridodialysis repair using 10 '0' proline suture

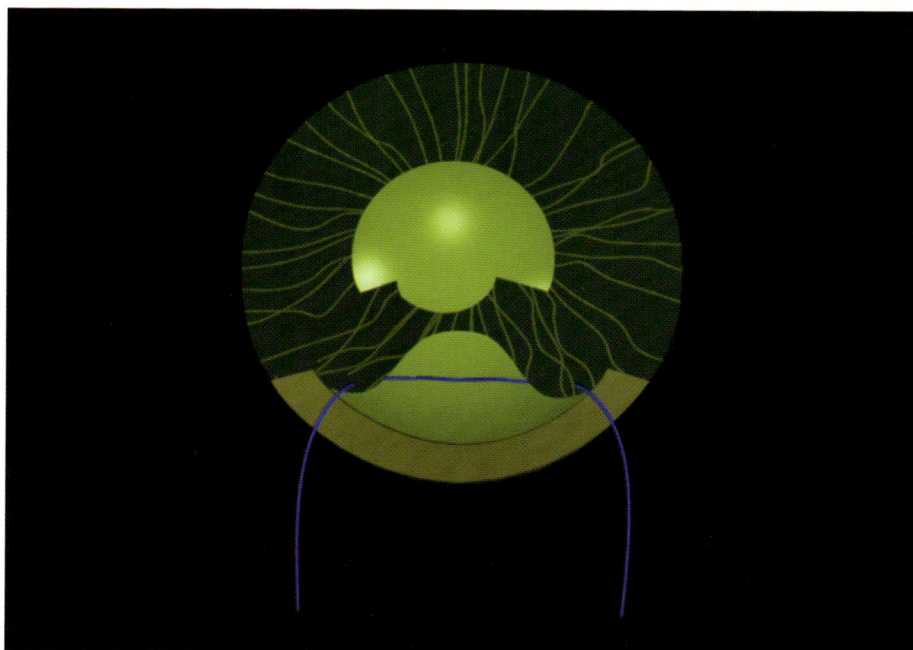

Fig. 31.3C: Suture passed through the two flaps of the dialysed iris and anchored to the sclera

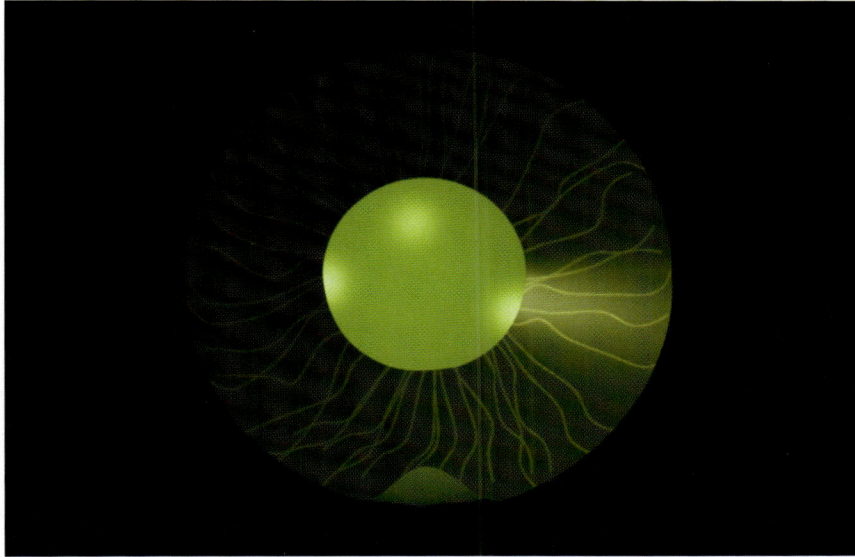

Fig. 31.3D: Completion of iris repair

In phaco surgery the phaco tip may cause damage to the Descemet's membrane or corneal endothelium or sometimes even the iris.

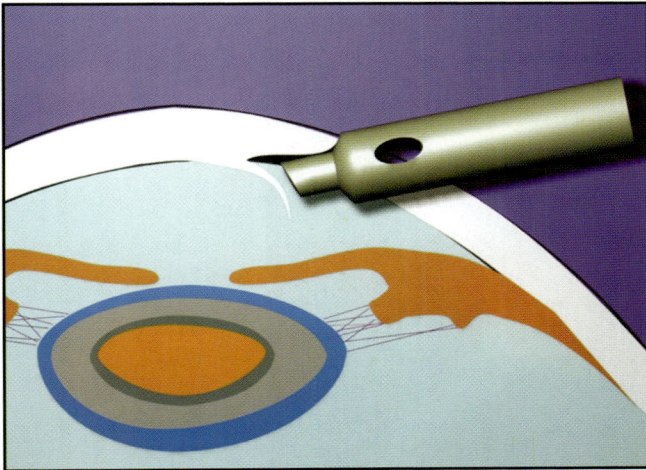

Fig. 31.4A: Descemet's detachment

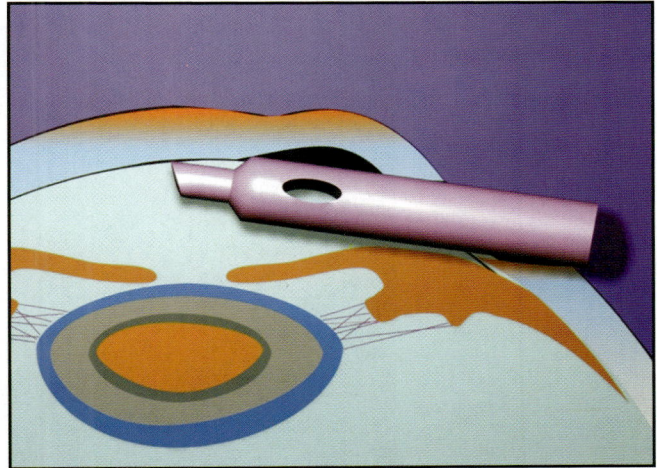

Fig. 31.4B: Corneal endothelial damage caused by phaco tip

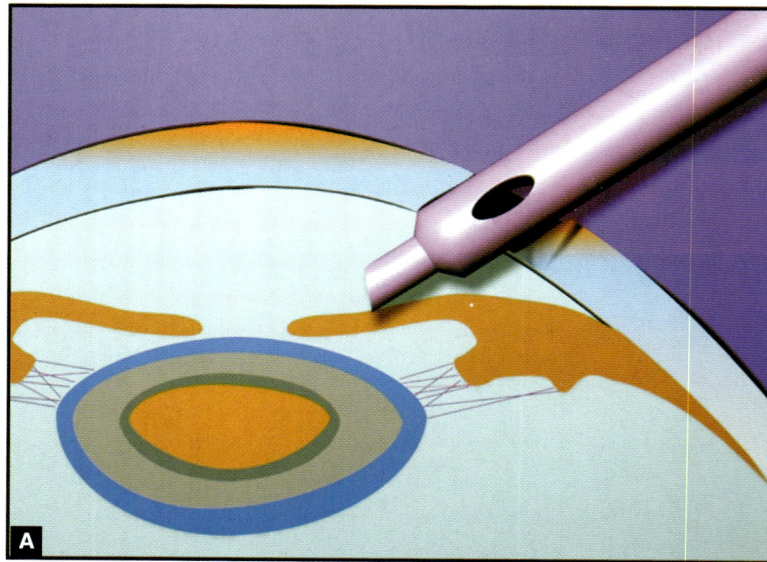

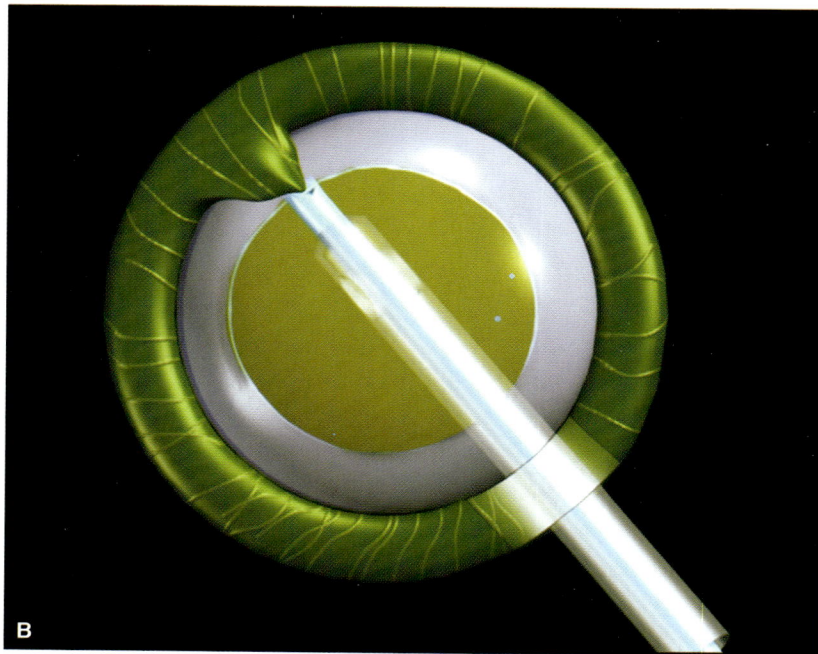

Figs 31.5A and B: Iris damage by phaco tip

- Tear of rhexis margin
- Zonular dehiscence
- Posterior capsular rupture (PCR).

Cortical clean up

May cause Corneal endothelial damage

Posterior capsule rupture may occur

Incomplete removal of cortex especially at 12 O' clock can be avoided by using a bimanual I and A.

IOL insertion

Corneal endothelial damage
  Zonule dehiscence and PC rupture may occur
  Damage to IOL optic or haptic may take place.

Expulsive Hemorrhage—Rare in SICS and Phaco

POSTERIOR CAPSULE RUPTURE (PCR)

Predisposing factors for PCR are :

1. Posterior polar cataract
2. Pediatric cataract
3. Raised intraocular and orbital pressures
4. Nuclear cataract
5. Hypermature cataract
6. Unco-operative patient
7. Proptosed eyes
8. Obese patients
9. PC rent in fellow eye
10. Improper anesthesia
11. Inadequate hypotony
12. Myopic eyes.

Predisposing factors for zonulolysis:

1. Aged persons
2. Intumescent cataract
3. Pseudoexfoliation
4. Hypermature cataract
5. Trauma
6. Marfans syndrome
7. Weill Marchesani syndrome
8. Microspherophakia
9. High myopes.

Factors predisposing to PCR during surgery:

1. Irregular capsulotomy
2. Traction on anterior capsular tags
3. Direct damage to the posterior capsule
4. Sudden collapse of AC
5. Excessive manipulation of capsule/nucleus during polishing
6. IOL insertion and dialing.

Danger signals of PCR:

1. Ring reflex
2. Radiating folds from center or from cannula

How to diagnose PCR:

1. Crescent reflex in zonular dehiscence
2. Irregular pupil
3. Irregular depth of AC

4. Wound gape
5. Difficulties in phaco/cortical aspiration.

Management of PCR:

Small rent – try to continue with same procedure or convert phaco into SICS.
   Place the posterior chamber IOL in the bag if possible or in the sulcus on the anterior capsule rhexis.
   Large rupture—perform a good anterior vitrectomy and Implant an ACIOL or a scleral fixated IOL.

How to avoid PC rents?

1. Adequate section
2. Adequate CCC
3. Gentle hydroprocedures
4. Usage of a good cannula
5. Avoid posterior pressure, blind procedures.

Management of Vitreous prolapse:

The following steps should be implemented—
1. Stop
2. Support
3. Extract
4. IOL
5. Vitrectomy

STOP

Whenever there is a vitreous prolapse, stop the procedure to avoid further complications.

SUPPORT

The posterior capsule is supported with viscoelastic,at the same time it will seal the dehiscence.

EXTRACT

The nucleus is extracted in the simplest way possible by converting phaco into manual small incision. If it is a small incision surgery,convert into conventional ECCE.

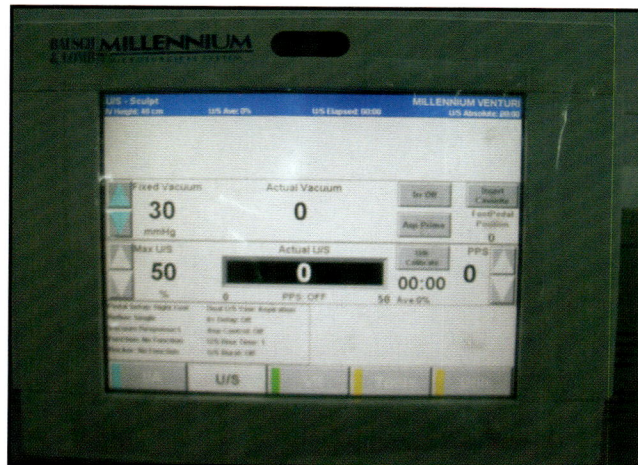

Fig. 31.6A: Vitrectomy machine (Bausch and Lomb)

IOL

IOL implantation is done depending on the capsular support. For example. PCIOL, ACIOL, SFIOL.

VITRECTOMY

Thorough anterior vitrectomy is performed both in front and behind the IOL. Care is taken such that the wounds are free of vitreous strands.

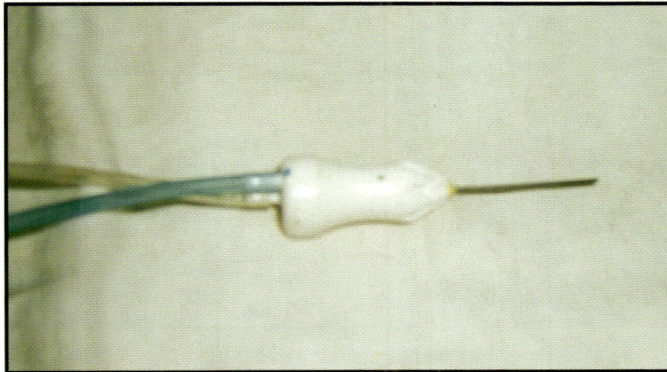

Fig. 31.6B: Vitrectomy cutter

POSTOPERATIVE complications

Immediate—Wound leak

Iris prolapse

Corneal edema and striate keratopathy

Hyphema

Post-operative uveitis

Secondary glaucoma

Dislocated IOL

Endophthalmitis

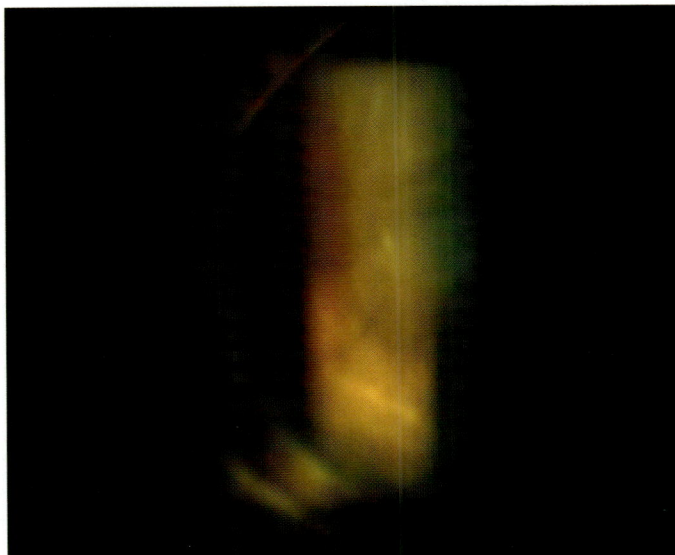

Fig. 31.7: Striate keratitis

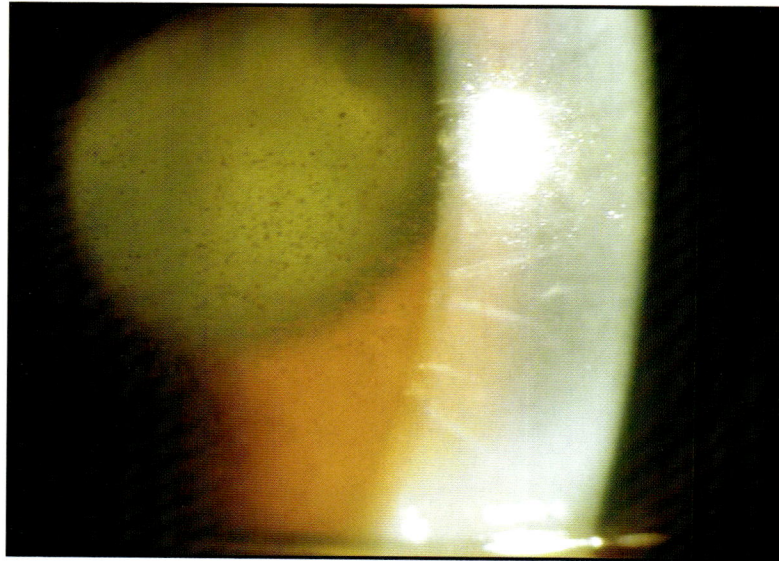

Fig. 31.8: Post-operative uveitis

Late: Corneal decompensation – bullous keratopathy

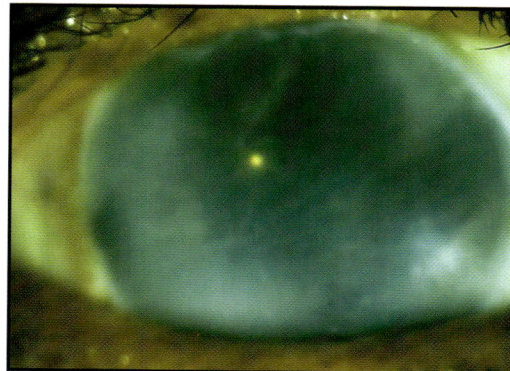

Fig. 31.9: Bullous keratopathy

Posterior capsular opacification (PCO)
Cystoid macular edema
Decentration of IOL
Retinal detachment
Late endophthalmitis.

CORNEAL EDEMA

Causes

1. Incomplete removal of visco
2. Retained lens matter
3. Improper IOL positioning
4. Intraoperative epithelial and endothelial damage
5. Vitreous in AC
6. Excessive phaco.

Management

Hypotensive agents
Hypertonic saline
Lubricants
Steroids.

POSTERIOR CAPSULAR OPACIFICATION

Causes

1. Proliferation of epithelial cells resulting in Soemmering's ring and Elschnig's pearls
2. Fibrosis of the capsule
3. Exudate or inflammatory membranes behind the IOL
4. Deposition of pigment or the ghost cells of the RBC
5. Remnants of lens material resulting in fibrosis.

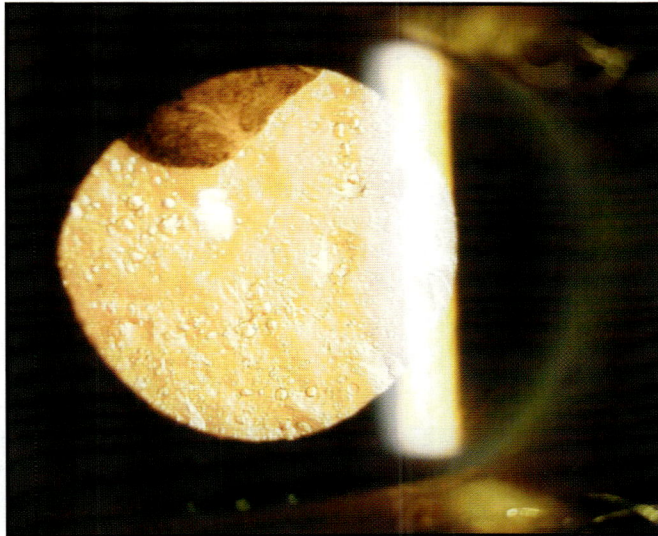

Fig. 31.10A: Posterior capsular opacification(Elschnig's pearls)

How to reduce Posterior capsular opacification?

1. Well centered   continuous curvilinear capsulorhexis(CCC)
2. CCC should be 0.5 mm less than size of optic so that it covers the anterior surface of the lens
3. Meticulous polishing of the capsule and thorough cleaning of the lens epithelial cells at the equator
4. Removal of the viscoelastic devices after the IOL implantation in the bag
5. Avoiding post-operative inflammation
6. Usage of square edge or optic edge IOL
7. Usage of biocompatible IOL. For example PMMA or Hydrophobic IOL.

Diagnosis

1. Visual acuity
2. Slit-lamp examination
3. Distant direct ophthalmoscopy (more accurate method).

Management

- Thorough dilated fundus examination is a prerequisite
- Posterior pole examination by slit-lamp biomicroscopy to rule out macular pathologies (CME, diabetic maculopathy, ARMD, small vein occlusion, etc) or optic disk pathologies (AION, glaucomatous optic atrophy)
- Indirect ophthalmoscopy is done to rule out any peripheral treatable lesions
- In case of a myopic eye check for the history, previous records and A-scan biometry findings
- If these reveal axial length greater than 26 mm Yag capsulotomy is contraindicated.

Treatment

- Adults
- Children
- Myopic eyes
- Eyes with retinal lesions.

Adult Eyes

1. Yag capsulotomy is to be started with minimal energy (1-2 mj)
2. Usually capsulotomy is generally achieved in 10 shots
3. A cruciate capsulotomy is created starting from mid periphery of one side and progressing to corresponding area on the opposite area
4. It must be insured that no free fragments fall into vitreous
5. Damage to lens and anterior vitreous must be avoided. This can be achieved by slight anterior defocusing
6. Post Yag treatment: Antiglaucoma therapy is to be started 2 hours prior to the procedure and to be continued till 4 days after the same
7. Apraclonidine eye drops is the drug of choice
8. Tablet acetazolamide is the second drug of choice
9. Topical; steroids are to be given up to 1 week after the procedure.

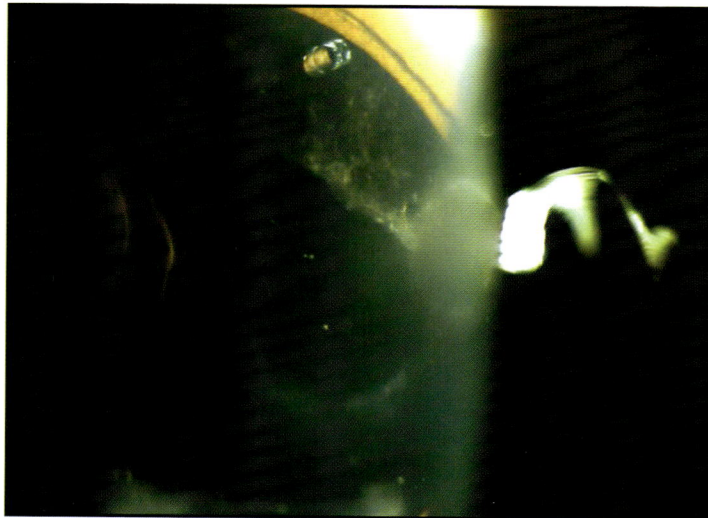

Fig. 31.10B: Yag capsulotomy

Children

1. Age up to 5 years: Primary posterior capsulotomy is preferred
2. In children above the age of 5 years YAG capsulotomy is preferred
3. In the presence of thick membrane, membranectomy with anterior vitrectomy is done.

Myopic eye

1. Polishing of capsule is preferred and YAG capsulotomy is avoided in high myopia as it may cause retinal detachment.

Retinal lesions

- First treat the retinal lesions
- Then attempt for capsulotomy with low energy and multiple spots
- If periphery is not visible due to capsular haze, post YAG fundus examination is essential.

ENDOPHTHALMITIS

Source of infection

- Irrigating solutions
- Viscoelastics
- Intraocular lens preserved in solutions
- Eye drops used before surgery
- Antiseptics used during surgery.

Air

- Air conditioning
- Respiratory system of the OT personnel
- OT air.

Patient

- Skin
- Lid margin
- Lacrimal sac
- Nasal cavity
- Previous surgeries like vitrectomy.

Surgeon

- Skin
- Respiratory system.

Instruments

- Improper sterilization
- Recycling of instruments
- Usage of same instruments for different cases as seen in camps
- Gloves
- Cotton swabs
- Bottles
- Phaco tips, tubings.

Clinical Features

Postoperative endophthalmitis should be suspected in the following conditions:
1. Patient complaints of disproportionate pain
2. Marked fall of vision.

Signs

1. Lid edema
   2. Conjunctival congestion with chemosis
   3. Corneal edema with or without ring infiltrates
   4. Wound dehiscence
   5. Hypopyon
   6. Loss of iris pattern
   7. Posterior synechiae
   8. Sluggishly reacting pupil
   9. Pupillary membrane.

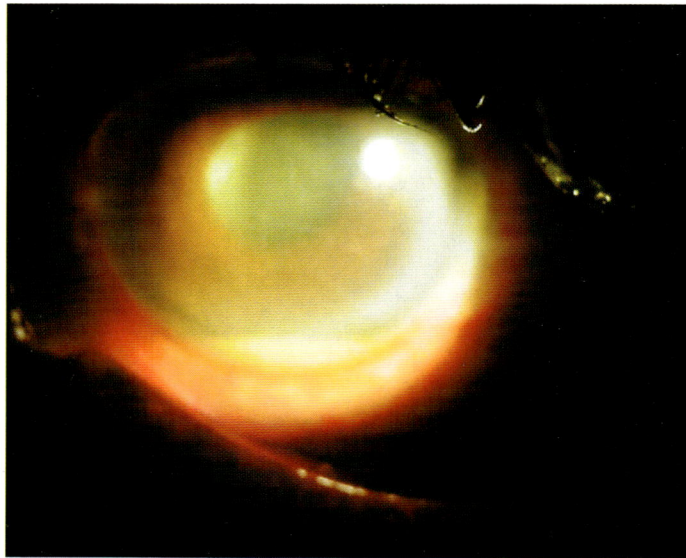

Fig. 31.11A: Post-operative endophthalmitis

Involvement of posterior segment is diagnosed by:
1. Loss of fundal glow (diagnosed by indirect ophthalmoscopy)
2. Vitreous white cells (Slit-lamp)
3. Thick exudates in the posterior vitreous (USG)

   The involvement of vitreous is a hallmark of endophthalmitis.

Confirmation of Diagnosis

1. Aqueous tap using 26 gauge needle
2. Vitreous biopsy using vitrectomy cutter.

   The sample so collected must be sent immediately for bacteriological culture.

Treatment

Intravitreal antibiotics are given through the Pars Plana route. The most commonly used antibiotics are vancomycin and ceftazidime.

Procedure

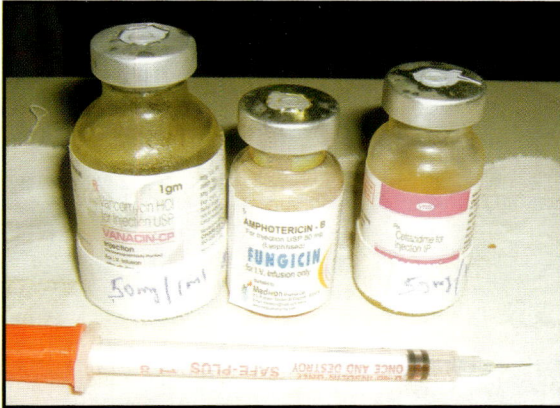

Fig. 31.11B: Intravitreal injections

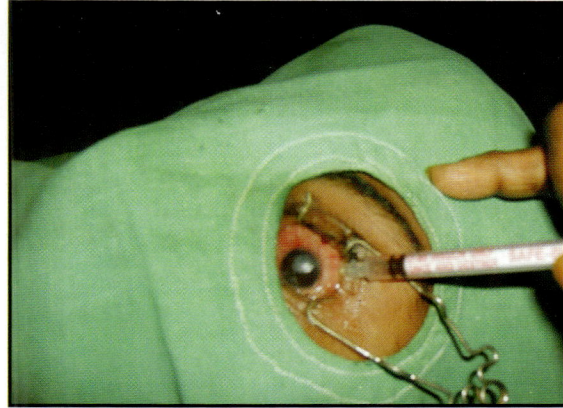

Fig. 31.11C: Intravitreal injection being given

1. Topical anesthetic should be instilled
2. IOP is recorded prior to the injection
3. In the event of the IOP being high, a few drops of aqueous are aspirated from the anterior chamber
4. 1 mg in 0.1 ml of vancomycin and 2.5 mg in 0.1 ml of ceftazidime is injected through the Pars plana (4mm from limbus) through separate entries as the drugs precipitate when used from the same port and same syringe
5. Subconjunctival vancomycin (25 mg in 0.5 ml) and ceftazidime (100 mg in 0.5 ml) are given separately.

How to prepare Intravitreal antibiotics?

1. 500 mg of vancomycin is diluted in the vial with 5 cc of distilled water (100 mg/ml)
2. 1 cc of this solution is taken in a 10 cc syringe and diluted with 9 cc of distilled water (10 mg/ml)
3. A insulin syringe (1 ml = 40 units) is taken and the above solution is drawn upto 4 units (0.1 ml) to get a final solution of 1 mg/0.1 ml
4. Similarly 500 mg of ceftazidime is diluted with 5 ml of distilled water in the vial (100 mg/ml)
5. 1 cc of this solution is diluted with 4 cc of distilled water in the 10 cc syringe (25 mg/ml)
6. 0.1 ml of the above solution is drawn in an insulin syringe (2.5 mg/0.1 ml).
   Along with Intravitreal antibiotics topical and systemic antibiotics are essential.

Vitrectomy

This has to be done by an experienced vitreoretinal surgeon.

When to perform vitrectomy?

1. Total absence of fundal glow
2. Inaccurate perception of light
3. Afferent pupillary defect
4. Corneal infiltrate
5. Infection with gram-negative organism
6. Patient worsening 24 hours after intravitreal injection.

Cystoid Macular Edema

It is the accumulation of fluid in the outer plexiform layer of the retina.

1. Incidence is higher with complicated cataract surgeries associated with posterior capsular rents and vitreous loss
2. 5-10 % patients undergoing ECCE have cystoid macular edema
3. 1 % of the patients undergoing phaco have cysoid macular edema
4. Majority of the cases are reversible.

Predisposing Factors

- Diabetic retinopathy
- Vascular occlusion
- Post-operative inflammations
- Drugs
  - Epinephrine
  - Latanoprost
  - Rifabutin.

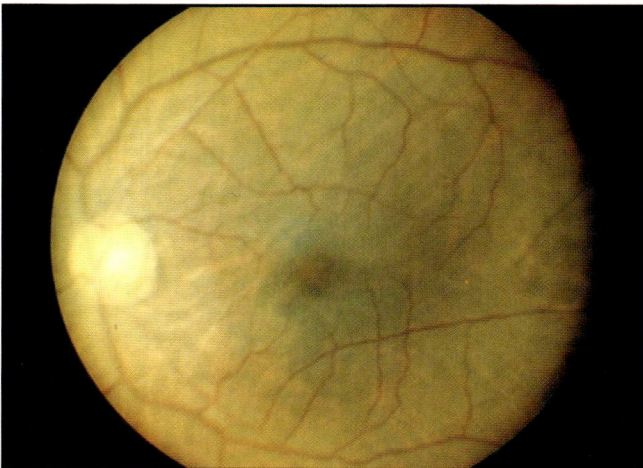

Fig. 31.12A: Fundus photograph

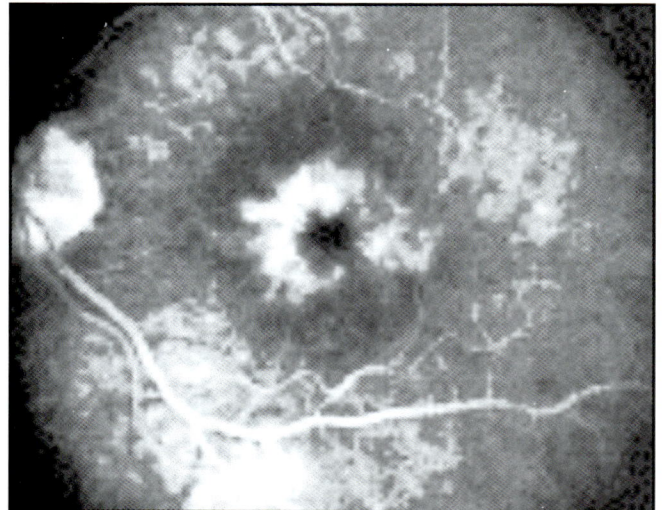

Fig. 31.12B: Fluorescein angiograph of cystoid macular edema of CME

Clinical Features

- Reduced visual acuity
- Metamorphopsia
- Symptoms usually present within 4 to 6 weeks post-operatively
- Late stages are associated with
  - Splinter hemorrhages
  - Foveal cyst
  - Lamellar hole
  - RPE mottling.

Treatment

Medical

- Spontaneous resolution

- Placebo
- NSAIDS
  - Topical
  - Oral
- Corticosteroids
  - Topical
  - Oral
  - Periocular
  - Intravitreal
  - Subtenon's
- Carbonic anhydrase inhibitors.

Surgical management

- YAG vitreolysis
- Vitrectomy
- IOL replacement
- Intravitreal triamcinolone.

Medicolegal issues

- Failure of diagnosis of CME
- Failure of diagnosis of associated conditions
- Use of newer drugs and techniques that are under trial like:
  - Hyperbaric oxygen
  - Retrobulbar injection of vasodilators
  - Somatostatin
  - Intravitreal bevacizumab.

32

Astigmatism and Cataract Surgery

Modern cataract surgery is not only for visual rehabilitation but for refractive surgery. The goal of refractive surgery is emmetropia. Astigmatism is one of the important factors to achieve this goal.

In cataract astigmatism maybe:

Pre existing astigmatism

Post-operative induced astigmatism

MANAGEMENT

Preoperative astigmatism

The amount of astigmatism and the meridian should be accurately measured before surgery by doing a good refraction.

Accurate keratometry (manual or automated)

Corneal Topography

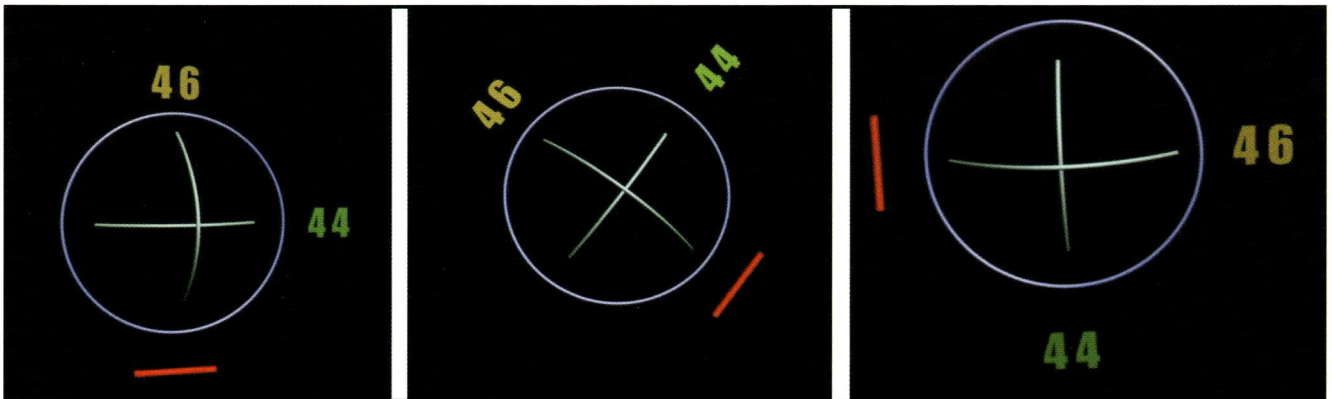

Fig 32.1A: Incision is taken along the steeper K meridian

Depending on the amount of astigmatism the management varies

0-1 D – Managed by the regular cataract incision in the meridian

1-2 D – Slightly longer incision in the steeper meridian

2-4 D – Regular cataract incision + astigmatic keratotomy 2LRIs

More than 4 D – Regular cataract incision + modification of IOL

power + astigmatic keratotomy – 2LRIs + CRIs

ASTIGMATIC KERATOTOMY

1. Corneal relaxing incisions (CRI)
2. Limbal relaxing incisions (LRI)

Corneal relaxing incisions

These were used to correct high degrees of astigmatism in cataract patients. The incisions are made concentric to the visual axis upto 90% thickness just outside the central optical zone(5.2 mm).

It usually causes overcorrection.

Patient may experience some problems like glare postoperatively as we go closer to the optical zone. They are no longer considered as a first line of management in dealing with astigmatism.

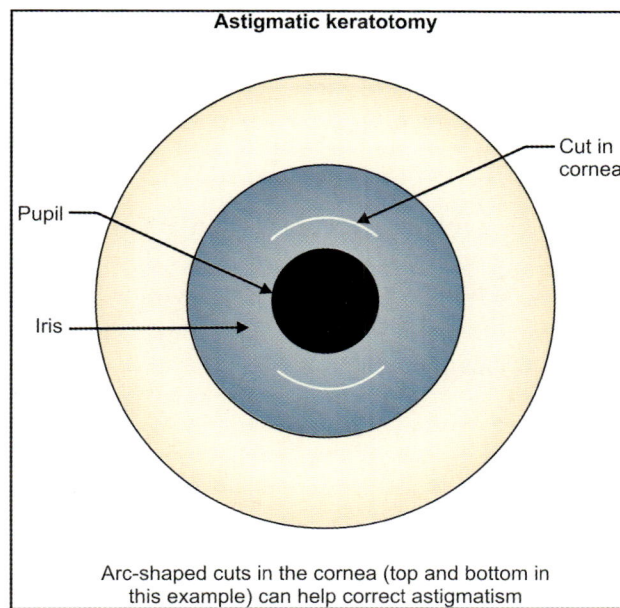

Astigmatic keratotomy

Pupil

Iris

Cut in cornea

Arc-shaped cuts in the cornea (top and bottom in this example) can help correct astigmatism

Fig. 32.1B: Astigmatic keratotomy corneal relaxing incisions

Limbal relaxing incisions

They are made close to the limbus just anterior to the palisades of Vogt. They are useful in correcting low to moderate astigmatism (Upto 3 D). They are easy to perform and do not cause post-operative glare.

LRI are made using a L320 micrometer knife. The number of incisions and length is determined depending on the amount of astigmatism.

LRI along with CRI can correct high astigmatism (up to 8D).

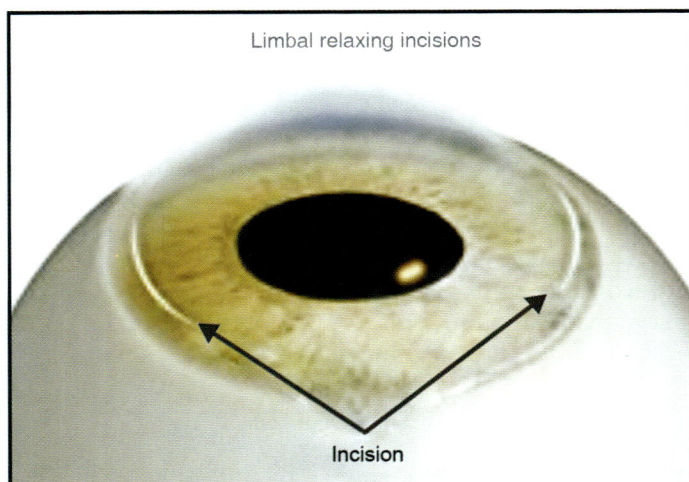

Fig. 32.1C: Astigmatic keratotomy Limbal relaxing incisions

Toric IOL

It is preferred in patients under 65 years with cataract and astigmatism. It is also used in any cataract patient with astigmatism greater than 3D. It is not widely used as it has disadvantage of rotation in the bag post-operatively losing its efficiency. Modern toric IOL (AICON) are relatively stable in the bag as they are made up of a hydrophobic acrylic.

Post-operative astigmatism management

1. Spectacles
2. Contact lens
3. Astigmatic surgery.

33

Anterior Chamber IOL

Whenever there is no sufficient capsular support, we have to resort either to anterior chamber intraocular lens or scleral fixated IOL.

Technically, the implantation of ACIOL is easier than scleral fixated IOL.

Characteristics of ACIOL

The overall diameter of ACIOL should be 0.5 to 1 mm larger than the horizontal visible iris diameter.

They have a 4 point fixation, smooth edges and a semi flexible nature with an anterior vault.

Indications:

1. Aphakia with no capsular support.
2. Accidental rupture of posterior capsule during cataract surgery.

   ACIOL is preferable in elderly. (Age > 40 years)

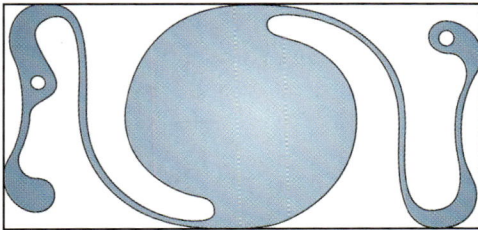

Fig. 33.1A: AC IOL

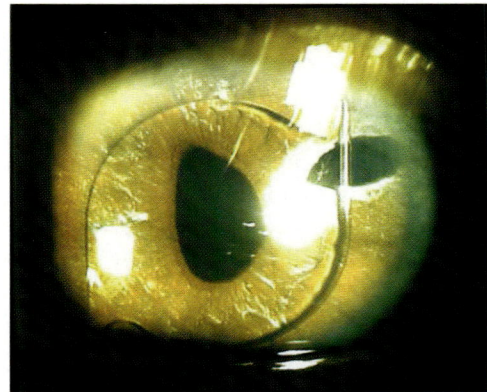

Fig. 33.1B: AC IOL implanted

Contraindications

1. Young patients (< 40 years)
2. Children
3. Pathology of anterior chamber structures like cornea (low endothelial count), angle and iris.

Procedure

Planned Surgery

Slit-lamp evaluation to know the intactness of anterior hyaloid face.

a.   If it is intact, preoperative pilocarpine is instilled and pupil is constricted as much as possible (pin point)

During surgery

Incision at right angles to original incision is preferable to avoid incisional complications and reduce cataract induced astigmatism.

Anterior chamber must be filled with cohesive viscoelastic and ACIOL should be implanted in proper position with the vault facing anteriorly. (It is to be noted that in PCIOL the vault faces posteriorly and in ACIOL it faces anteriorly. Hence dialing of ACIOL is anticlockwise and that of PCIOL is clockwise) .

Lens haptic should be placed at right angles to incision so that the loop will not erode through the fresh wound.

Advantage of cohesive viscoelastic is that, it can be removed en masse. Even if mixed up with vitreous, there is no inflammatory response. In the absence of cohesive viscoelastic, air can be used.

b.   When vitreous is in AC

Here the anterior vitrectomy with bimanual cutters is mandatory.

Avoid performing vitrectomy manually and using coaxial cutters.

Do not hydrate the vitreous.

A thorough anterior vitrectomy is the secret of a successful ACIOL Implantation.

After the vitrectomy the anterior chamber is filled with air or cohesive viscoelastic (Healon) and ACIOL is implanted as described before.

If the eye is hypotonic, wound may be closed with 10-0 nylon.

ACIOL with intraoperative rupture of PC or zonule

If vitrectomy equipment is available, an attempt for primary implantation of ACIOL is made. If not well equipped, close the wound and refer the patient to a center where such facilities are available.

During surgery dry vitrectomy should be performed without hydrating vitreous. If hydration occurs, more and more vitreous loss occurs. The end point of vitrectomy is a round pupil, no strands of vitreous in the section and formation of a deep anterior chamber.

At the end, air bubble or cohesive viscoelastic is put into anterior chamber and IOL is implant.

Care should be taken not to leave any lens matter in the periphery or in vitreous.

If necessary intraoperative intracameral pilocarpine(without preservative) can be used to constrict the pupil.

PBI is a must in all cases of ACIOL implantation.

Complications

1.   Corneal edema
2.   Uveitis
3.   Glaucoma
4.   Loop erosion from the wound
5.   Malpositioning
6.   CME.

34

Secondary IOL Implantation

Indications

Aphakia is the common factor in all the indications. The various indications are:
1. Spectacle intolerance
2. Contact lens intolerance
3. Prevention of amblyopia and fusional problems
4. External disease (vernal kerato conjunctivitis, eczema, lid margin diseases)
5. Legal and occupational standards–example vehicle driving.

Preoperative Evaluation

1. Best corrected visual acuity
2. Slit-lamp examination—
   • To assess the anterior segment, i.e. anterior chamber angle, cornea, iris and vitreous
   • To plan the type of IOL
3. Orthoptic assessment to assess the chance of post-operative diplopia using contact lens in unilateral aphakics.
4. Assessment of preoperative cylindrical power and its axis.
5. Assessment of fundus by direct and indirect ophthalmoscopy
6. A-scan biometry to assess the intraocular lens power
7. Ultrasound B-scan, when fundus is not visible due to membrane in the pupillary area.

Types of Secondary IOL

1. Anterior chamber IOL(ACIOL)
2. Posterior chamber IOL(PCIOL)
3. Scleral fixated IOL(SFIOL)
4. Iris fixated IOL

Anterior Chamber IOL(ACIOL): Implantation of ACIOL is described in the chapter 33.

Posterior chamber IOL (PCIOL): It is preferable to fix the lens in the bag wherever possible by carefully dissecting the capsule using viscoelastic and avoiding the loss of vitreous. In case of difficulty, the lens can be implanted in the sulcus.

Key Point
• Check the position of IOL all the time in case of doubt, use SFIOL and tie atleast one of the loops to the Sclera.
• A thorough vitrectomy is performed. No vitreous should be present anterior to the lens or in the wound.

Scleral Fixated IOL (SFIOL)

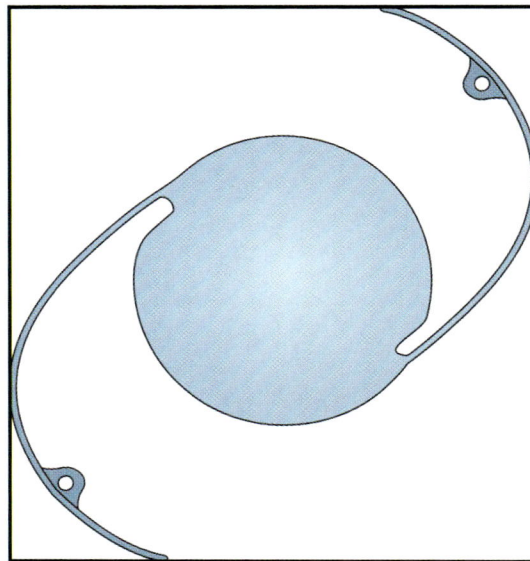

Fig. 34.1B: Scleral fixated IOL

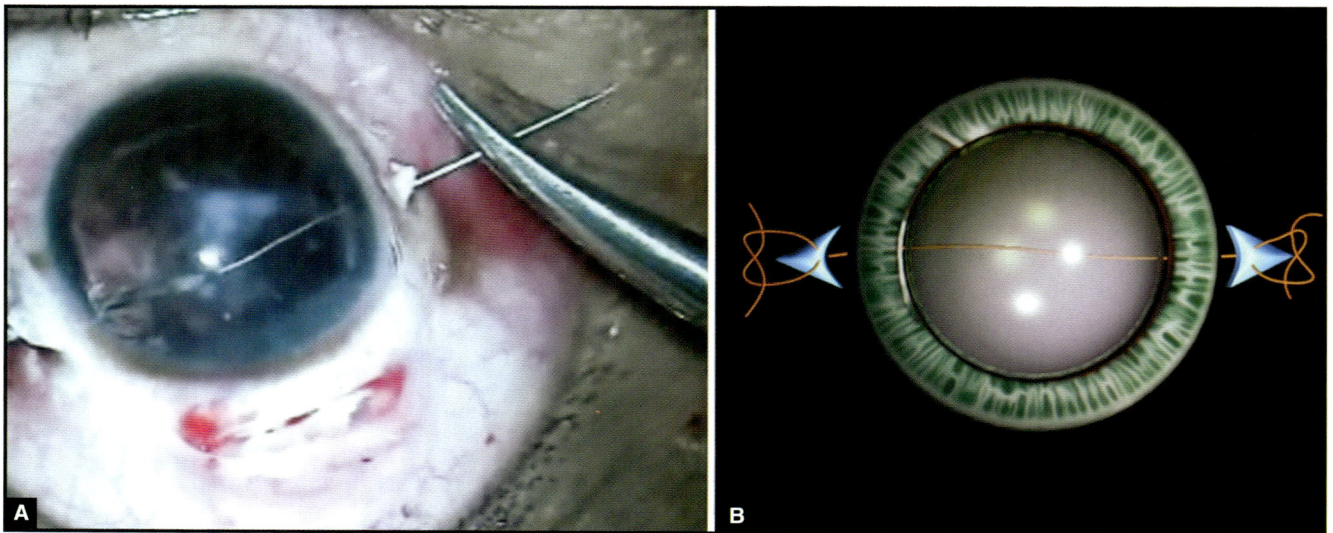

Figs 34.2A and B: Passing a proline suture

In the absence of total capsular support, it is preferable to place a SFIOL. In this procedure 10-0 prolene with long straight needles are used. The first step is to make a triangular partial thickness flap(3 mm long), similar to the fashion that is attempted for a case of trabeculectomy at diametrically opposite (i.e, 180° apart) positions. Through one end, a 26 gauge needle is passed into the posterior chamber. Through the other end, a straight needle with prolene is passed into the lumen of the 26 gauge needle. The 26 gauge needle is slowly withdrawn ensuring that the straight needle comes out along with it.

A 6.5 mm tunnel incision is created at right angles to the suture line. The suture loop is taken out externally through the tunnel using the Sinskey's hook. The loop is cut and the 2 free ends are tied to the eyelets provided on each haptic of SFIOL.A cohesive Viscoelastic or air is used to protect the endothelium and maintain the Anterior Chamber. The Lens is inserted and dialed to the proper position. Both the ends of the suture are pulled ensuring the proper centration of IOL.

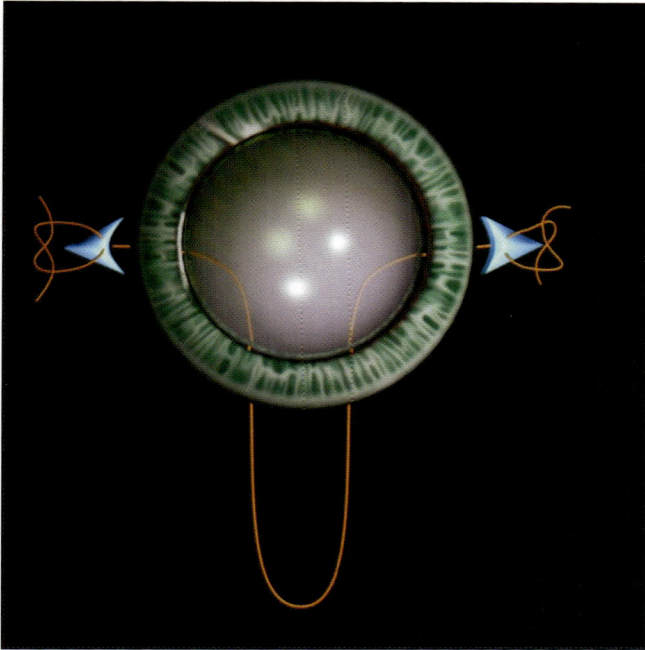

Fig. 34.2C: Suture is drawn out as two end of loop at 12 o' clock position

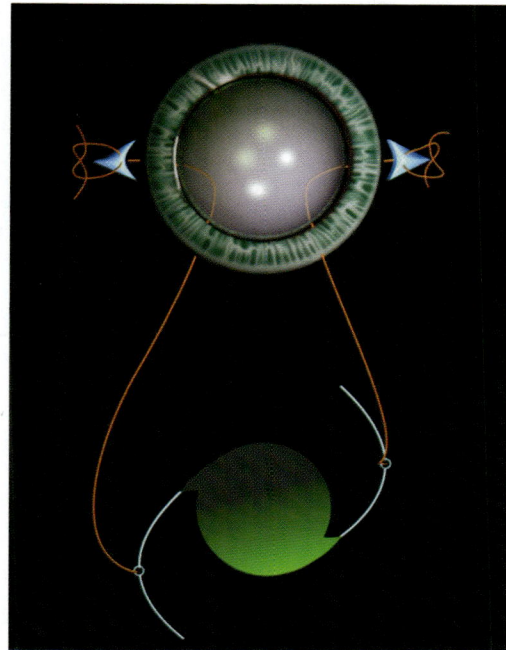

Fig. 34 .2D: The loop is cut and they are anchored to the eyelets of scleral fixated IOL

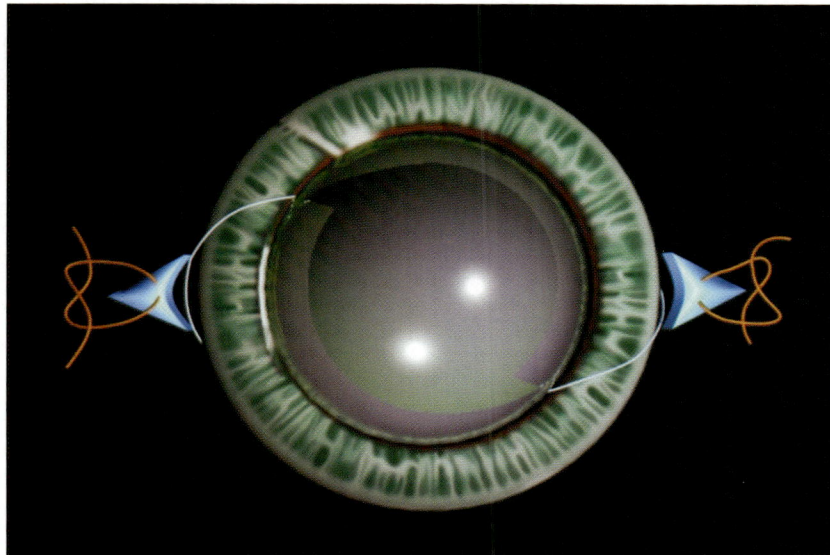

Fig. 34 .2E: IOL is kept in position and the suture is anchored to the sclera at 3 and 9 O' clock

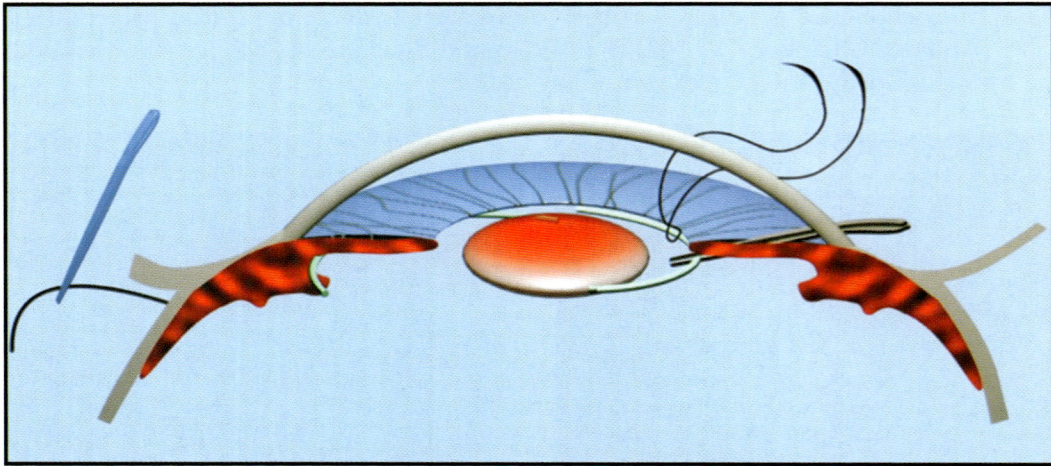

Fig. 34.2F: IOL in position and anchored to the sclera

The sutures are then tied in the triangular scleral bed. The scleral flap is then closed using single 10-0 suture at the apex.

2 side port entries are made into the anterior chamber using MVR blade. The remnants of the vitreous anterior to the lens and in the section are cleaned using high cutting rate and low aspiration. The anterior chamber is maintained at the end by injecting either saline or air.The side ports are closed by hydrating the cornea.

In case of hypotony, the tunnel is closed using horizontal or 'X' sutures.

Iris Fixated IOL

It is indicated in the event of subluxation of PCIOL where one or two loops haptic are fixed to the iris.

It is indicated during penetrating keratoplasty where the globe is hypotonic and it is not feasible to place SFIOL where the lens is fixed to iris either by using the dialing holes for the suture or by fixing the haptic to the iris by sutures.

In case of decentred SFIOL, an additional iris fixation will help in centering the IOL.

Complications

* Post-operative uveitis
* Retinal detachment
* Cystoid macular edema
* Glaucoma
* Fusional difficulties
* Corneal decompensation.

Index